Vegan Diet Meal Plan for Beginners 2020

2 Books in 1: Vegan Keto Diet Meal Plan and Intermittent Fasting 16/8. The Best, Most Efficient and Proven Way to Change your Body, Image and Life

Paty Breads

<u>INTERMITTENT FASTING 16/8</u>

<u>VEGAN KETO DIET MEAL PLAN</u>

Paty Breads

Intermittent Fasting 16/8

The 16/8 method as the best option to lose weight, regenerate your body, increase your energy, control your hunger and feel better. A step-by-step guide to change your image and your lifestyle

Paty Breads

Furthermore, the information that can be found within the pages described forthwith shall be considered both accurate and truthful when it comes to the recounting of facts. As such, any use, correct or incorrect, of the provided information will render the Publisher free of responsibility as to the actions taken outside of their direct purview. Regardless, there are zero scenarios where the original author or the Publisher can be deemed liable in any fashion for any damages or hardships that may result from any of the information discussed herein.

Additionally, the information in the following pages is intended only for informational purposes and should thus be thought of as universal. As befitting its nature, it is presented without assurance regarding its prolonged validity or interim quality. Trademarks that are mentioned are done without written consent and can in no way be considered an endorsement from the trademark holder.

Table of Contents

Maintain Discipline

Patience Pays

Have a Clear Mind

Effective Reliability

Confidence

Resetting

Productivity

Rest

Tips to Help You Sleep Well

Get Enough Sunlight

Avoid Watching Before You Go to Bed

Dark Sleep

Quality Is Not Quantity

Power

Stay Strong

Try to Avoid Your Temptation.

Prepare Your Refrigerator to Make Fasting Days Easier.

Remember That Social Meeting Does Not Have to Be Included in Food.

If You Are a Sanitizer, Stay Away from the Triggers.

Reward Yourself

Learn to Tell the Difference Between Hunger and Other Emotions.

Conclusion

Introduction

Fasting doesn't mean not eating; it's about eating with planning. It's a way to plan your meals so you can benefit more. Intermittent fasting involves changing the way you eat but not the kinds of foods you eat.

Well, in particular, it's the best way to treat it without eating crazy foods or lowering your calories for nothing. Most times you will try to keep your calories the same when you start a non-stop fast. (Most people eat large meals over a short period.) Besides, intermittent fasting is a good way to control muscle mass, where they rise in the stomach. All this said the main reason people try to fast is fasting. We will discuss how intermittent fasting happens to get fat in a minute.

You need to understand that intermitted fasting is a strategy that you can use with ease and succeed in your endeavors. You do not have to opt to lift bad weights while maintaining good weight because it requires very little behavioral change. This is a good thing because it means that the fasting sequence falls into the category "simple and easy that you will do, but well enough that it can make a great difference. Have you tried various ways to get yourself in good shape only to end up disappointed? This book is critical to you because it contains all the information that you need to achieve your health goals. If you want to reduce weight, then you can be sure to get such benefits if you read and comprehend the information contained in this book. Let's get started!

Chapter 1: The Problem with Modern Diet

What Are Issues with Modern Diet?

We all know we need to eat healthily. We also know that we need to limit how much soda, drinks, processed foods, sugar we eat. But even though we know these things, it doesn't mean they are easy to follow.

According to a recent Food and Health Survey conducted by Psychology Today, 52 percent of Americans believe it is easier to calculate their taxes than know how to eat healthily. Too many people are having problems with this modern tax code, which means that many people have trouble figuring out how to eat the right foods for them.

We live in a country that is battling obesity. More than one-third of people in the United States are considered obese, and many are also considered to be overweight. However, these statistics do not show the full picture. Three out of three adults are considered overweight or obese, meaning that most people will fall into this category.

Why are these statistics so bad? Many factors contribute to obesity. One major culprit is classic American food. There has been a significant decline in the quality of our food as we have gone from a nation dependent on food from local farms to a nation that produces most of the food. This transition has increased our appetite for food because it is available now.

Also, many readily available and easily consumed foods are high in fat, sugar, and calories. All of these things help increase weight. From the sugary snacks, we get from the restroom to all the food chains around us, the quality of the food, and the amount we eat have dramatically changed. We can eat healthy foods without stopping if we want to, which is why obesity is so prevalent in our culture.

The first thing to look at is the amount of food we eat. The number of calories everyone needs may vary from person to person. Ingredients include your genes, your level of activity, your overall health, height, age, and gender. However, the target number used in food labels is about 2000 calories per day. This number is already fairly high for those living a stable life. It is also possible to eat 2000 calories or more in one sitting if you go out to eat.

Although the food out quickly us pushing the number of calories, it is also possible to eat too much when I eat at home. It is important to learn how to start eating what we need to work on, rather than eating because something tastes good, or we get bored, or tired.

To calculate the average daily calories consumed by Americans, organizations are examining the amount of food available per capita that shows the amount of food consumed. In the United States, this ends up around 3800 calories per day. Even when you take into account the fact that some of these foods are lost or discarded daily rather than eaten, the average American consumes 2700 calories per day. This is the approach that everyone will need, even if they lead an active lifestyle and not many Americans.

Now, we need to also discuss the quality of food most Americans eat. Growing up, most of us learn from our parents and teachers about what is good and what is not. Fruits and vegetables are seen as such well, and sugar and sweets are bad. The rest of the diet may not be as good as before, but they were good in moderation. Although we have been taught about healthy eating at an early age, it is still culturally difficult to follow these tips.

According to the Agricultural Department in the U.S., the top six sources of calories for most Americans are fruit-based sweets, yeast, poultry, sports/energy drinks, and alcoholic beverages. Remember that healthy fruits and vegetables are not listed. In the top five lists, the most common foods Americans eat are refined fruits and sugar. It is estimated that only 8% of the average American diet consists of fruits and vegetables.

According to a study by the US Department of Agriculture (USDA) in 2010, nuts, meat, and eggs make up 21% of these foods; oils and fats make up 23%, and calorie sweeteners make up 15%. Food that is not good for us constitutes 61 percent of our diet.

The time of day we eat is also important. Most Americans live a busy lifestyle and do not have time to sit and eat a balanced diet. In effect, they eat walking, usually in some areas unhealthy, or eat at night when their metabolism is slow. Besides, many Americans are sitting in bed and eating unhealthy snacks while watching television. Sometimes the diet is high, so we eat non-stop food.

It is important to learn the steps necessary to limit the amount of food we take each day. It is tempting to eat readily available foods. But, if you want to get back to your health and get better in a good way, it is important to stay away from classic American food and choose something good for you.

When you hear fasting, you can think of people who go for weeks without eating for religious reasons. You may think it is unhealthy or incapable of doing it because you love food. But intermittent fasting is different from religious fasting, although they share common ideas.

Indirect fasting is limiting your calorie intake in parts of the day or not eating too much on certain days. Your body still gets the nutrients it needs, but you eat fewer calories, so keeping it simple gravity. Some of the various types of fast cot will have discussed later in this book.

The reason this diet is successful is that it is effective in reducing the amount of fat in your body, as well as the number of calories you eat. Since you are reducing the time allowed to eat or reduce your calorie intake during certain days of the week, it is easy to lower your total calorie count. You can also choose how much time you would like to do quickly. Some people choose to do it for a month or more while others may fit their lifestyle, so they stick to it in the long run.

Avoid Unhealthy Eating Habits

After dinner, you are overweight, but you can't resist ordering desserts. If your stomach is hungry all day, then sweeten yourself until you fall asleep. Or maybe you can always eat something, such as walking, parking, or driving.

If any of these situations seem common, you can use your eating habits in preparation. They can all show unhealthy habits and can lose weight successfully for a long time.

Listen to Your Body

Anyone struggling with food allergies will develop a disruptive behavior that nutritionists can call. Poor eating habits can take many forms, from eating poorly to developing obesity and eating disorders, bulimia, or anorexia.

To allow yourself to want to lose weight and develop a healthy diet, your first step should be to accept your body and be proud that you are a member of a Weight Loss Program to keep your body healthy.

One of the best ways to regulate your eating habits is to stay active - learn how to eat when you are hungry and stop smoking after eating. It is easy to say, but with a little education, you will learn how to control your calories but not feel lost.

No One Is Perfect

Your goal should be to remain neutral, not perfect. Do not have physical cravings for food that can lead to physical inactivity, which can lead to many stomach ailments and eating disorders.

This book will help you improve your diet and create a diet plan that includes your favorite foods, including low-fat or healthy foods, to keep you healthy and satisfied. You need to slowly change your diet and improve your lifestyle to get the best results.

One powerful example to avoid eating is to put away a lot of calories from your face. Resistance is impossible when the food is under your nose!

But don't give up. You do not have to resist the urge to enter. What to do is to prevent parties and places with lots of junk food. Before you begin your first meal, please do a "stomach test": are you hungry, or do you just crave for something to eat?

If the food is like putting some oil in a container, our lives will be easier, but eating is more than an empty container.

Many cultural, behavioral, emotional, social, and environmental factors can help us determine how much time we spend in the stress of the job, and such hard experiences can make us start eating.
Consider whether you decide to eat or not, rather than decide without being conscious or unconscious. Can you choose what to eat? It will be easier if you start choosing a healthy diet - you will

have to regain the spirit as you experience the benefits of your tradition.

How to Change Bad Habits

Change is not always easy, especially for long-term behavior. So here are some tips to help you put away these bad habits into practice:

- Develop a plan to manage your daily contact with them. Decide how to address your weaknesses to be aware of the situation.

- Replace unhealthy foods with good food. If eating at night is your weakness, please give yourself a small snack in the evening.

- Too much sleep - it can slow down your eating time!

- Reduce TV viewing. You don't have time to try meals, and you have time to exercise.

- Set goals that are realistic for you. Not sure what will happen to you. Slowly change your habit of taking drugs.

- Thinking positive, negative thoughts like "I can't" or "I'm tired and distracted" can enable you to succeed in your course. Write inspirational ideas and read them when you need help to focus on your goals.

- Find your friends or hire supportive friends to maximize your chances of success. Studies have shown that support is essential to the success of behavioral changes and barriers.

Brush Your Teeth After Dinner to Reduce the Temptation to Eat

Foods buy organic foods (or personalized foods) that you can combine with fruit. The package that makes up the economy supports investing.

Wait at least ten minutes before seeking a second help to give your stomach time to express your thoughts. Eat your day with breakfast. According to one study, when most people eat calories in the morning, their total daily intake is less than calories in the evening.

Chapter 2: Intermitted Fasting, What Is It?

What does the actual meaning of fasting mean? Almost all of us know the word fast. The reasons people quickly differ are from one group to another. For some people, it is a religious tradition; they sacrifice to pray. Others have no reason to; they just eat food. In early societies, people used to go to the woods to work and to eat while they rest.

Temporary fasting is not part of the fasting practices described above. It is not a religious tradition, nor does it drive without time and no food - it is an option. It is best described as a diet pattern that changes during meal times and fasting periods, with each season running at a fixed time. For example, in the 16:8 type, you fast 16 hours and 8 hours when you can eat.

Note that it is not food but a form of eating. Less is said about the foods you should eat, but more emphasis is placed on eating. Does this mean you can eat anything you want? The truth is you mat eat what you want. Like everything else in life, you will need to get out of what you are into. Eating clean is one of the three factors in the success of a successful diet. Does this mean you live with chicken and broccoli? We are human beings and believe in enjoying life, but as you already know, moderation is the key here.

It is important to note that IF is not a program that is out of place, will change over time, and disappear like most weight loss programs. It has been around for a long time and has been popular for many years (even now you are learning it). It is one of the first health and fitness changes in the world today, and it is recommended by a variety of health and fitness experts.

Intermittent Fasting History

When you compare the traditional "diet," fasting is easier and less stressful. It is always done. You know that you will be conscious every time you don't eat breakfast or dinner. Historically, our ancestors were fasting during the hunting season.

Once the field is established, civilization will follow. If there is not enough food or season, people will fast without problems. Cities and fortresses process cereals and meat in the winter. Before watering, no rain means famine. People should store food for as long as possible before fasting until the rain returns, and the crop can be revived.

Religion develops in this way of living together, sharing, and spreading beliefs and customs. Religion also records fasting. Hindus call it "Vaasa" and designate special days or holidays, using personal pens or commemorating their gods. Islam and

Judaism have Ramadan and Yom Kippur, which is a place where work, food, clothes, and love are forbidden. In the Catholic Church, fast six weeks before Easter or Holy Week.

Fasting Science

Modern agriculture and the "food" industry (or food-like things) have completely changed the way people view or eat food every day, leading to the laundry list that today's society faces. IF is an ancient tradition, and the science behind its health benefits will soon be available to the public. When fasting, you can basically make your body clean, repair, and restore its best function.

The three main health promotion methods associated with fasting include biological metabolic control, glandular dysfunction, and various lifestyles.

Circadian Rhythm Biology

Humans (and other organisms) have evolved into biological clocks that produce circadian rhythms to ensure that your body functions work in a negative time throughout the day.

They occur in a 24-hour light-dark cycle and are affected by biological and behavioral changes.

Body fluid consumption can negatively affect metabolism, which may lead to being overweight and diseases like cancer, heart disease, and type 2 diabetes.

This Is a Place for Temporary Fasting.

Eating symptoms seems to be the main time for how your body works and regulates metabolism, physiology, and behavioral ways that contribute to your overall health and well-being.

Certain behavioral interventions, such as (you guessed it!) indirect fasting, can promote the synthesis of circadian rhythms, leading to gene expression, metabolism, and changes in hormones and weight control, all of which play an important role in your health result.

Microbiome of the Gut Microbiome

The gastrointestinal tract (GI), also known as the intestine, plays a very important role in regulating multiple processes in the body.

Many bowel movements (and almost all physical and biological activities in the body) are affected by the above-mentioned circadian rhythm.

For example, gastric emptying during the day, blood flow and glucose metabolism are more frequent than at night.
Therefore, chronic obstructive pulmonary edema may affect bowel function, leading to an increased risk of poor metabolism and chronic disease.

The gut microbiome, also known as our "second brain," has become a broad target for health and disease research because of its wide participation in the body's metabolism, physiology, nutrition, and prevention.

Direct fasting has a direct and positive impact on the disease microbiome:

Slow down

- Insufficient system structure
- Promote energy balance by strengthening self-esteem
- With a great understanding of the potential for disease prevention and treatment, research on bowel and fasting is still emerging.

Life Behavior

Intermittent fasting has been shown to alter various health behaviors such as calorie intake (e.g., how much you eat), energy expenditure (when you are exercising), and sleep.

No wonder these three factors are one of the biggest factors in fasting today: losing weight.

A recent study showed that increasing the fasting time at night to more than 14 hours resulted in a significant reduction in calorie intake and weight gain due to:

- Energy level
- Sleep satisfaction
- Sleep restrictions

Intermittent fasting also reduces nighttime eating, which leads to poor sleep quality and reduced sleep time, leading to increased insulin resistance and obesity, diabetes, heart disease, and cancer.

The next question you might encounter is why you should consider fasting first. Humans have experienced fasting for many years. Sometimes they do this because it is necessary because they can't afford anything. Then there is time to fast for religious reasons. Religions such as Buddhism, Christianity, and Islam advocate some form of fasting. Fasting is also normal when you are sick.

Although fasting sometimes has a negative meaning, fasting does not have any natural meaning. Our bodies are better able to cope with the time we should not eat. Many things in the body change when we are fasting. This will help our body stay active during the drought.

When we fast, we find a significant decrease in insulin and blood sugar levels, and also an improved increase in Human Growth Hormone. Although it was done in the early stages of food shortages, it was used to help people lose weight. Burning fat becomes lighter, easier, and more effective.
Some people decide to go faster because it helps their metabolism. This fasting is good for correcting various health problems. There is also evidence that regular fasting can help you live longer. Studies have shown that these mice live longer in the fasting zone.

Other studies have shown that fasting can prevent various diseases such as Alzheimer's disease, cancer, type 2 diabetes, and heart disease. Then some people choose to go faster because it suits their lifestyle. Fasting is helpful for life. For example, the less food you have to do, the easier it will be to live.

Why Do You Want to Fast?

Intermittent fasting is a practice of diet planning so that your body can get the most out of it. Fasting is a simple, sensible, and healthy way to promote weight loss, rather than reducing calorie intake by eliminating all your favorite foods or maintaining a normal diet. There are many ways to fast, but it is defined as a specific diet. This model focuses on the transformations you make while eating, not what you eat.

When you start with an intermittent fast, you are likely to keep your calories the same, but instead of spreading your food throughout the day, you will eat larger meals over a shorter period. For example, instead of eating 3 to 4 meals a day, you can eat one large meal at 11 am, and then another large meal at 6 pm, with no food between 11 am and 6 pm, and 6 -After the evening, eat until 11 am. This is one way of fasting, and others will be discussed in this book in later chapters. However, you must first understand why this method works.

Intermittent fasting is a method used by many bodybuilders, athletes, and members of the body to gain muscle mass and percentage of body fat low. It's a simple strategy that allows you to eat your favorite foods while still promoting fat loss and muscle gain or maintenance. Endless fasting can be applied in a short or long time, but the best results come from adopting this lifestyle in your daily life.

While the word "fasting" can intimidate the average person, indirect fasting does not mean that your soul is hungry. To understand the managers behind the successful transition zone, we first go through the two digestive regions of the region: the feeding region and the fasting region. Three to five hours after eating, your body is in what is called the "fed state." During the feeding phase, your insulin levels increase to absorb and balance your diet. With increased insulin levels, it is not easy for the body to burn fast. Insulin is a hormone produced by the pancreas to regulate the levels of glucose in the blood. Despite its purpose for regulating, insulin is technically a storage hormone. When your insulin levels are high, your body burns your food for energy rather than your stored fat, which is why increased levels prevent weight loss.

After three to five hours are full, your body has completed the meal preparation, and you enter the recovery state. The condition behind absorption lasts from 8 to 12 hours. This time the difference is when your body enters the fasting state. Since your body has completely processed your diet at this time, your insulin levels are low, making the stored fat more likely to burn. Fasting state, your body does not have the energy left to eat, so reserves are burned. Regular fasting allows your body to achieve the fat-burning rate that you would normally achieve on an average, 'three meals a day' mode of eating. This alone is why many people experience immediate results without intermittent fasting without even altering their physical activity while eating, or eating. They simply change the timing and the way they eat.

When you start the program for fast and relentless, it may take some time to leave things out. Don't be discouraged! If you change, get back to the fast mode when you can. Avoid hitting yourself or feeling guilty. Negative self-esteem goes a long way in getting back into your shape. Making a lifestyle change takes a conscious effort, and no one expects to do it right away. Unless it is known that you are going for a long time. Since when you eat, fast and relentless you will take some time to learn. As soon as you choose the right course for you, focus and be positive, you will find your place in no time.

Unlike some of the other meal plans, you may have to continue; fasting will work. It uses your body and how it works to its advantage to help you lose weight. It's easy to hear some fear when fasting. You can assume that you need to live for days and weeks without eating (and being able to put off their diet for a long time even when they want to lose weight), and it will be difficult for you.

Fasting endless slightly different from the one you think you can. Not only is it really difficult to fast for weeks at a time, but it is also not good for the body. Your body will often go into a state of hunger if you eventually fast. It will take you to spend a lot of time without eating so the body will work to save calories and help you keep up with fat and calories as long as possible. This means you will not only be hungry but also lose weight.

You do not have to worry about how fast fasting will work in the process of starvation. Fasting is effective because you will not be fasting until the body gets into this state of hunger and stops losing weight. In hindsight, it makes fasting long enough for you to be able to speed up your metabolism.

With a temporary fast, you will find that when you go for a few hours without eating (usually no more than 24 hours), the body will not go straight into the hunger process. Instead, it wants to eliminate available calories. If you ate the right amount of calories during the day, the body will return to eating until it consumes the stored fat deposits and uses it as fuel. Likewise, when you follow a series of fasting plans, you force your body to burn more fat without putting in any extra work.

Here are some quick tips for success:

First and foremost, you mustn't expect to see results from your new lifestyle immediately. In effect, you need to plan on doing the task at least 30 days before you start judging the results correctly. Second, it is important to keep in mind that the quality of the food you put into your body is still important as it only takes a few quick meals to finish all your hard work. Finally, for the best results, you will need to incorporate a simple exercise routine during the fasting days and a more gentle exercise on full-calorie days.

Intermittent Fasting Types

Several major types of intermittent fasting are there that you can choose to follow. These Somalis can all be effective, and the one that suits you will depend on your preferences, your schedule, and your lifestyle. Some of the fasting options you can go with include:

- Method 16/8: This will ask you to fast 16 hours daily and eat for the other 8 hours. So, you can choose to eat only from noon until 8 pm or after 10 pm. You can choose one of your favorite eight-hour windows.

- Eat-Eat: In a week, it could be twice or once when you will not consume anything from the first day to the next. This gives you a 24-hour fast but still allows you to eat every day of your fast.

- 5: 2: You will choose two days of the week to fast. During those two days, you are only allowed to have up to 500-600 calories per day.

Of course, there are differences between the three above. For example, some people decide to limit their even bigger windows by eating only four hours and fasting for this fast. Most people who fast this fast choose to follow the 16/8 method because it is the easiest to adapt and will give you great results along the way. The fasting is simple and effective. It helps you to limit the calories you eat and burn more fats and calories than you normally feed.

Chapter 3: How Do You Fast?

One thing that many people like about interactive fasting is that it can offer you many options. As I mentioned, there are several different ways you can do a quick fix based on your schedule and lifestyle. Some people find that they have a few busy days during the week and so those days will fast. Others like the idea of reducing their eating window and doing fasting every day.

The fasting method you choose is yours. They can all be very effective and will give you some of the benefits you are looking for. Let's look at some of the fasting options you can go with, so you can choose the one that is right for you.

The 16:8 Method

There are different ways to learn IF. However, they all have the same meaning; all are in seasonal feeding and fasting.

- The time to fast – it depends on the time length in different methods. During this time, you have not eaten at all or zero-calorie drinks.

- Feeding time – also varies with the length of time in each method. During this time, you can eat whatever you want moderately to avoid too many drinks. It is advisable to eat normally and do not look like compensation during your lack of food. Some features like Warrior Diet may require you to eat foods in a particular way.

Before we look at the 16: 8 method, it is important to point out that temporary fasting is not for everyone. Below are some of the people who can't try the temporary fast:

- Under People under 18 years
- People with diabetes (both type 1 and 2) without seeing a doctor first
- Mothers Pregnant and lactating mothers
- People with Eating Disorders
- People with low body fat
- People with high cortisol levels

WARNING: Before you do any diet, exercise program or your usual changes should go to a doctor or other relevant professional.

Now let's look at the 16: 8 method in particular.

16:8 Schedule

As the name implies, this method is divided into two periods; for 16 hours of fasting and 8 hours of feeding time. It is important to monitor your feeding time regularly. This means that you cannot decide to eat from 8 am to 4 pm today and change from 8 pm to 4 am the next day. This is designed to create a schedule that is easy for your body to adapt to and easy to follow. Remember, the hungry hormones are released concerning eating habits? Changing your routine regularly will make you hungry all the time and experience a problem with these hormones.

This method is said to be durable and easy to stick to as you are not required to live without food for a long time, and can easily adapt to the lives of most people in everyday life. For example, the average person sleeps for eight hours. You only need to fast for an additional 8 hours while you are awake, making the fasting period shorter.

For example, if your last meal was at 10 pm, you would fast until 2 pm the next day, and some would sleep, while others would be busy - you won't know exactly when. This method is popular as you can still have dinner with your family or friends before your feeding window closes. Important note: Some research suggests eating late at night produces higher insulin than daytime affects sleep quality and enhances nighttime storage.

Factors to Consider for Achieving Success

Goal Setting

I recommend that you have a clear view of what you want to achieve. Not as many goals as I want to get - "fit," "healthy," or "lose two pounds" just won't cut it when it's hard. You need a clear reason to do this, or you are likely to quit. When I train a client, I tell them to consider 3 things.

What do you want to do that you cannot currently attend?

- 30 days
- 90 days
- 12 Months

What do you want to look like?

- 30 days
- 90 days
- 12 Months

How do you want to feel?

- 30 days
- 90 days
- 12 Months

When they complete this, I also tell them to ask themselves why they want these things and what they think will be different from these goals. This will help you identify what matters to you. Many times our goals originate from external influences, but at the end of the day, they should be right for you. Analyze your data and set:

- Day Goal
- Day Goal
- Month Goal

Collection

Evaluate your schedule! I always see people who choose only the dining window, so I have time to eat during this time. Not a good start! Also, assess where you might struggle to go without food. For example, if you are a lazy mocker it is not wise to set your fasting window during the slowest part of your day. If eating dinner with your family is a tradition, then allow your dining window. Be smart when choosing a feeder window. Make this task as easy as possible for yourself.

Support

It is important to surround yourself with good people on the same journey. It will be difficult, and in some cases, you will need to stop. Finding other people to support you is the key to success and can be the difference between quitting and continuing!

Maintain Discipline

Of all the things you can find in the world, discipline is one of the most valuable. Discipline is the most important factor you need to have long-term success. Even though you may be fasting and losing weight, there is a huge burden on discipline because you have to actively train your mind and not want the body's diet. In most cases, people allow their physical desires to take over and make their own decisions.

When you fast, you actively seek discipline to make sure you do not let your body make the decisions for you.

When you can continue discipline, this has an impact on your entire life. When you choose to urinate on what you love, this will eventually lead to your demise.

Patience Pays

It is often proved that patience is good. When you can be patient, you can endure and weather any difficult situation with the knowledge that you will overcome the other.

The opposite of a sick person is that of angry anger. Anger is usually associated with children. Importantly, an adult can be easily seen as an adult because when they do not find their way quickly, they throw a fit.

When you are working toward a goal like stress, there will be some negatives involved. This does not mean that you will never be able to be satisfied. It means you can't have an item right away.

When you can actively participate in the rejection of yourself temporarily because of a specific goal, you will be able to apply that virtue to other aspects of your life.

Have a Clear Mind

In many cases, people share the power of fasting with the evidence of their minds. Many people go through stress and anxiety. When you can get rid of these points, this will help you to focus specifically. This is because you have no fog associated with the brain.

When your mind is clear, you will be able to think in a way that is physically perfect for what you want.

When your mind is stressed with anxiety, you will make decisions that are not always the best. Those decisions do not reflect what you want deeply because fear affects you.

When your mind is clear, you eliminate issues like fear, anxiety, and depression.

Understand the power of the mind. Wherever your mind goes, your life will follow. When you can prove something, you will be able to have a completely different experience but with more power.

Effective Reliability

For centuries, fasting has been recognized as a major component of certain religious groups. It is famous for Islam, Judaism, and Christianity. Most people who practice fasting practice at certain times of the year (Ramadan, Rent, etc.). At these times, they eliminate something they especially want (food, TV, social media) to focus their attention on God.

When deciding to fast weight loss purposes, you may feel a little bit different. However, if you maintain a spiritual belief in a higher power, this will affect that relationship. This is because you may be able to rely on something superior to help you withstand your body tests.

This culture is especially good for people who are emotionally eating to cope with their emotions. When you do not have the food you have in your hands, this forces you to rely on the higher power (religious or not) to get the strength you need to overcome difficult times.

Confidence

In most cases, people do not allow themselves to develop the strength that is really within them.

- When you can work out your self-denial fasting, this is a confidence boost.
- When you can check out something on your list of activities that is difficult, this will make you feel good about yourself and your abilities.
- When you know you can overcome something difficult, this changes the way you view yourself.

It also affects how you view future challenges. When you can overcome a challenge, it gives you the confidence to continue. When you feel mentally strong, this will affect your ability to look at the situation rather than the situation, and you will come out with the challenge.

Resetting

There are times when people are constantly eating and not having time to give up. When you fast for weight loss, this is a good opportunity to get rehab.

You are allowed to clean your system and get rid of any problems. This is not just physical. This is from a psychological and spiritual perspective, as well.

If you like proverbial resettlement, many people do the same when the holidays are over. During the holidays, people eat and drink because it is a popular season. However, it may not common for individuals to have an overwhelming feeling after it is over.

This is one of the main reasons people start weight loss trips as a New Year's resolution. For many, it is an attempt to repair or delay the process.

Productivity

There are many different types of articles, videos, and all where people like to discuss life create more productive. Maintaining high levels of productivity is to achieve great success in the eyes of many. While this may not be important to everyone, many people believe this.

As a result, many people are looking for ways to increase their productivity to make them feel successful. If you would like to enjoy the added benefit of fasting, understand that productivity can fall under this umbrella. This is mainly because production can be a clear product.

When you are focused and do not have the burden of stress on your brain, this naturally increases your ability to produce more. Consider how you feel after eating Thanksgiving. In most cases, people return to tiredness and the length of the bed near you. While the body takes time to digest all these foods, it will spend more energy on your efforts to complete other tasks. As a result, people are slow and want to sleep.

If you fast, your body does not spend as much energy to digest it except water. As a result, you have more energy to engage in other activities.

Rest

One of the benefits of fasting for weight loss is the ability to relax and relax. When your mind is clear, and you will not be dealing with too much stress, this will help you remain in a state of mind for a long time. So, when you sleep, it will be easier for you to avoid falling asleep.

This is great news for people struggling with insomnia or sleep issues. As you develop a nighttime routine and are in the middle of fasting, your body will be able to turn around and have an easy time getting quality rest.

Tips to Help You Sleep Well

Get Enough Sunlight

Our body system or "body clock" plays an important role in producing hormones. This is strongly influenced by sunlight. Stevenson explained that Light, especially sunlight, signals your glands and organs to be the time to wake up, waiting in line to produce the hormones of the day (often helping you stay alert and awake). If our body receives less sunlight and more light in the morning (such as televisions, laptops, and smartphones), our circadian clock will rise. This can cause our glands to produce hormones that prevent them from falling asleep. Poor quality of sleep hinders the production of hormones such as HGH and can even stimulate the production of hormones such as insulin. If that happens, we will not burn fat at night!

Avoid Watching Before You Go to Bed

If you are watching TV until 11 pm or sleeping on your phone, the quickest way to improve sleep is to stop using your device at least an hour before bedtime. Remember how our body clock affects sunlight? It is also influenced by artificial light. Our eyes are great light sensors, and the blue light emitted by our favorite screen stimulates our body to produce day-to-day hormones and primarily makes us awake and active. For these bad boys in our body, insomnia will be difficult, and our bodies will not produce the anabolic hormones we need to repair and lose weight. Some of Stevenson's evidence only came out in the dark. Have fun!

Some people often argue that watching television or other device helps them sleep without being distracted. The above information is to achieve quality sleep, and although you may feel it, I find it in most cases, this is because the client has made it a habit. I encourage you to find other activities to change your equipment, rather than lying in the dark about worrying about not going to sleep.

Dark Sleep

While this may seem obvious after the first two tips, some people forget this guide when they were not told. We cannot control outdoor lights, such as traffic lights and disturbing safety lights, but these can still affect our sleep at the molecular level, interrupting maintenance, and making us tired the next day. Leave your windows with heavy curtains to stop the fog outside of the lights that are damaging your healing process!

Quality Is Not Quantity

One of the most useful points I have come across in Stevenson's book is that there is a window of sweet time during the night where sleep is the most effective. During this window, our body produces the highest number of hormones needed for repair and fat loss. He explained that this was about 10 pm to 2 am and clock out the window. He also noted that this can vary depending on the time of year and the time you are in, but he advised that you get to bed as soon as possible after dark.

Improving your sleep habits is the key to weight loss, muscle building, and living a healthier life in general. This important ingredient is often overlooked in weight loss programs and maybe the remaining part you need! Proper sleep will ensure the adaptation of the essential hormone to fat-burning maybe even more important than increasing your exercise habits. Set a regular bedtime and make sure you lie in bed about 30 to 60 minutes ahead.

Power

When you have power, you have resilience. When you endure, nothing can stop your path. The advantages of fasting to lose weight include your ability to improve. When you are working on developing talent, it is a good idea to start small.

Think about fasting for specific hours a day. So, as you manage those goals, build on that for many hours. A long time ago, you will be able to do three days of fasting without much difficulty. When you can fast for a long time, this will increase endurance and ability.

Stay Strong

One of the reasons people love superheroes is because of their strength. They can force them when they need to achieve a goal.

Although the superheroes of their weakness, they can find ways of overcoming. When you can fast for weight loss and lose weight, this will allow you to develop an inner strength that you can apply to your spiritual, personal, and professional life.

No matter, know that it has many benefits for fasting. Don't trust the hype when people say that fasting is dangerous.

When you do it right, it can directly impact your entire life and make you a better person. Even though you are fasting for weight loss, your mind and body will improve your life significantly.

Try to Avoid Your Temptation.

One thing that may hinder your efforts on fasting days is the temptation of other foods in your cupboard. If you are fairly sensitive to visual experimenting with food, you may need to shop every few days instead of shopping every week or two. It can also help if you have family members or someone who lives with you and will not follow Fasting.

Prepare Your Refrigerator to Make Fasting Days Easier.

Try to place your food on the fasting day on the refrigerator shelf. This can help train your eyes (and your mind) that only those foods are available on fasting days. Eventually, you may find that your eyes are not wandering around in the fridge, looking at foods you can't eat.

Remember That Social Meeting Does Not Have to Be Included in Food.

Eating out can be a big part of your social life. Sharing a good meal or several drinks with friends and family is part of our culture. However, there are many other things you can do to enjoy the fasting days that do not involve eating. Focusing on these activities will help keep your mind away from food but will ensure that you do not become a vet when fasting. Invite some friends to go to a tennis game, take an art show, spend a day at the beach, or sign up for a dance class with a bill.

If You Are a Sanitizer, Stay Away from the Triggers.

Many of us have stimulants, except at mealtimes or hunger, which shows us to eat. Time off work can be automatically sent to us by a vending machine. Watching TV can be adapted to mealtimes. You may want to bring the leftovers to your children when you clean the dishes. Spend some time before your meal is listed at mealtimes, and then make a plan to deal with these triggers while eating. Take time off from work and have the opportunity to take a ten-minute walk. Allow other family members to clean the plates after dinner. Make work needles, cut cards or cabbage, do some extension, or chew gum when you are watching television.

Reward Yourself

The best way to achieve a great goal is to set a few small ones and celebrate them as they have achieved them. For any of the days of fasting completed or any lost pounds, treat yourself a little. It can be weights, a new book, an evening out with you and your husband, or just an hour to yourself.

Learn to Tell the Difference Between Hunger and Other Emotions.

Most of us eat junk food. We eat because we are angry, we eat because we are not lazy, or we eat because we are tired. Begin writing down your feelings when you are thinking about taking a snack. You may find that most of the time, you just need to move, talk on the phone with a friend, or go to sleep.

If you feel hungry, drink water.

It is often difficult to tell the difference between thirst and hunger. Each time you feel a craving for a snack, drink a glass of water. You may find that hunger pangs often disappear.

Other Ways of Intermittent Fasting

Diet 5:2

Another option you can go with is the 5:2 diet. This one asks you to eat in a normal manner for five days of the week with the discipline to limit yourself to no more than 600 calories the other two days. This is sometimes called the "fasting" as well.

Nowadays fast, it is recommended that women should stay at 500 calories and 600 calories for men. For example, you will eat normally every day of the week, and on Monday and Thursday, you will only eat two small meals for a total of 500-600 calories. You can choose any day of the week like the days of fasting until you do not put them back. Choose the two busiest days of the week and do your fasting.

There aren't many studies out there about the 5:2 diet, but since it's fast, it will give you the many benefits you are looking for. You will be able to do it without having to worry about making food all day.

Eat a Regular Diet

Diet-Eating requires you to avoid eating 24 hours once or twice a week. This model was first published by Brad Pilon and was a popular way to do it consistently over a while. It is possible to fast in the fast while still eating one meal a day. Most people eat dinner after day and do not eat until after dinner the next day. This will allow you to never go for a whole day without eating but fail during the 24-hour drinking period.

You can change this however you like. If you find it easier to skip breakfast or lunch or lunch to lunch, then you can choose one of these options. During your fasting, you are allowed to have coffee, water, and other calorie-free beverages to satisfy yourself, but you are not allowed to have any food at all.

Remember that you only fast for one or two days a week. When it is time to eat normally, you need to eat the same food that you would have if you were not fasting. This will help you lose weight without damaging your body.

The main issue of continuing such a fast is the 24-hour fast is difficult for most people. However, you can easily. You may find that starting with a fast, such as a 16-hour fast, can give you better results, and then you can start fasting longer. Going all day without eating can be difficult, and most people choose to follow one of the other fasting options to see the same results.

Another Fasting Day

With this option, you will be fasting every other day. There are several options you can go with, and it will depend on what works for your needs. Some fasting allows you to have around

500 calories in your fasting days. You will find that most laboratory studies about the transition zone used some form of fasting day to assist in determining all the health benefits.

Fasting every other day can be difficult for most people. Forcing you to fast every other day can be a challenge. Fasting every other day is something you will need to build on. You are likely to feel hungry several times a week for fasting, and it is difficult to cope in the long run.

Worrier Food

This is another popular option that you can choose from during non-stop fasting. It involves eating small quantities of raw fruits and vegetables during the day, followed by plenty of evening meals. This requires you to fast throughout the day, to eat enough to satisfy, and to eat in the four-hour window at night.

This food is one of the first foods to incorporate some kind of indirect fasting. Such diets also include food choices similar to Paleo food. You will not fast most of the day and night celebrations, but you will be eating a diet full of foods that look like what you can discover in nature.

Skipping Meals Spontaneously

You can try this if you want to prepare your body for a temporary fast or if you don't want to worry too much when eating. In this zone, you do not need to worry about following one of the more structured fasting plans. From time to time, you will skip meals. You can do this when you are hungry or when you are busy and not eating. It is a great myth that you have to eat every hour to avoid starvation.

The body adapts well to dealing with a long time without eating. It lacks a number of foods, especially if you are not hungry or busy; it does not harm your body. Every time you skip a meal or two, you do it technically. If you are too busy to have breakfast at the door, make sure you eat a healthy lunch and dinner. If you miss work assignments and are unable to find a place to eat, then it is okay to miss out on food. This is not harmful, and it really helps to save time.

You may not see good results compared to some of the other options, but it is better than nothing and easy to work with. You may try to skip a meal or two during the week and lose some weight when it works. As you can see, there are many different options that you can work with when you are ready to go fasting. Some of these will be easier than others, and some may fit your schedule better. You will need to choose the fastest way to work in your daily life.

Chapter 4: Why Should You Do Intermittent Fasting?

There are various plans for meals that you can choose. Some will help you limit your carbon intake and focus on good fats and protein. Some will limit your fat intake and focus on a healthy, healthy scourge.

With all the options on the market and a few of them being legitimate weight loss options, you need to know why you need to be fast and uninterrupted. This unit will look at the various benefits of direct fasting and how it will change your health.

It Modulates the Cells, Hormones and Genes Function

The failure to eat for a while leads to certain things happening to the body. For instance, it will start to regulate cell function and change some of your hormone levels, making it easier for body fat to enter. Other changes that may occur in the body include:

- Levels of insulin: insulin levels will decline slightly, which makes it easier for the body to burn fat.

- Human Growth Hormone: Growth hormone blood level can significantly increase. High levels of this hormone can help build muscle and burn fat.
- Cell Repair: The body will begin the process of repairing the cells, such as removing the waste from all the cells
- Genetic profiling: Some beneficial mutations occur in several genes that will help you live longer and protect against disease.

Weight Loss and Body Fat

Many people go fast in succession to lose weight. In most cases, indirect fasting will naturally help you eat less. You will end up consuming fewer calories, which will lead to weight loss. Besides, fasting strengthens the hormone to facilitate weight loss. Low growth hormone and insulin levels help your body break down fat and use energy. This is why short-term fasting can increase your metabolism by at least three percent.

On the one hand, it boosts your metabolism to burn more calories while also reducing the amount you eat. According to a review that was released in 2014concerning the scientific studies of intermittent fasting, people were able to lose up to 8 percent of their body weight in less than 24 weeks.

It Helps with Diabetes

Type 2 diabetes is a disease that has become popular in recent years. Anything that could lower the resistance of insulin could also be useful in lowering the blood sugar levels hence protecting you from type 2 diabetes.

According to some researches on Intermittent Fasting, there was a reduction of blood sugar from three to six percent, while insulin was reduced by 21 percent and 31 percent. A study carried on rats that were diabetic also proved that Intermittent Fasting could be crucial in the protection of rats from kidney damage; a common challenge for diabetics. This suggests that indirect fasting may be a good option for people at high risk for type 2 diabetes.

Simplifying Life

While this may not be considered a health benefit like any other, it is still important to note. Many people find that temporary fasting can make life easier. They know that they need to have a focus on to eat, as long as they are allowed to eat for hours. They can go a few days a week without having to worry about eating. Overall, this meal plan can make your life easier.

When you can cut down on some of the work you need to do during the day and focus on something else, you may end up worrying about your life. We all know that stress can hurt our health and our lives. When you can reduce stress, it is easy to be the healthiest version of yourself.

Good on the Heart

Heart disease is considered to be the world's largest killer. Intermittent fasting can help with some of these risk factors, such as low blood sugar levels, inflammatory markers, blood triglycerides, cholesterol, and high blood pressure. The main issue is that many studies on intermittent fasting have been conducted in animals. We need to do more studies that test fasting and human heart health.

Can Help with Cancer

Many people get cancer every year. This disease can lead to extreme conditions, and its characteristics include cells growing in an uncontrolled manner. Fasting is something that is said to be having great benefits in terms of your metabolism, which can lead to a reduction in cancer risk. Some human studies show that fasting cancer patients have been able to alleviate some of the chemical side effects.

Good on the Mind

Something considered to be working for the physical body could also work for the brain? Fasting can help improve the metabolic symptoms that are common in helping the brain stay healthy as well. This may include helping with insulin resistance, lowering blood sugar levels, reduced inflammation, and chemical stress.

There have been several studies conducted in rats showing how intermittent fasting can contribute to the growth of nerve cells, which improves brain function. Fasting can also help to increase the levels of brain activity that arise. When the brain is deficient in this, it can cause depression as well as other mental issues.

It Helps to Improve Cells

When we move fast, human cells can begin to be called the "resistance" of the digestive process. This involves breaking down the cells and metabolizing any proteins that are no longer used. As self-medication increases, it can help prevent human illnesses like cancer and Alzheimer's disease.

May Prevent Alzheimer's Disease

Alzheimer's is a neurological disease that has become common nowadays. The disease is not curable, and to ensure you are safe from it, prevention is better than cure. According to a particular study which was contacted on rats, one of the ways to prevent the disease is through intermittent fasting.

There are some cases whereby findings suggest that if you include fasting on a daily basis can have a positive impact when it comes to dealing with Alzheimer's disease. The studies have been done to both animals and human beings. Apart from this disease the studies also indicate that intermittent fasting can help in the prevention of other diseases like Parkinson's and Huntington diseases

Some case reports indicate that lifestyle changes (including daily or at least short-term fasting) help improve the symptoms of Alzheimer's disease in nine of the 10 patients. Animal studies have also shown that this fasting can help prevent other neurological diseases such as Huntington's disease and Parkinson's disease.

Although most of these studies were done on animals, the results seemed promising. Temporary fasting is a trend, and research on its mechanisms for good health is not new. It takes time to learn all the benefits of fasting.

Regular Fasting Can Help You Live Longer

One of the most interesting things about interactive fasting is that it can help you live longer. Several studies in rodents have shown how intermittent fasting can help extend their lifespan—similar to what happens when you gradually reach the regular calorie limit. In some studies, the effect was surprisingly low. One is that animals that fast every day live 83% more than those that do not.

While it is difficult to justify an increase in its lifespan due to the intermittent fasting still has not been conducted in research on long-term populations to determine this, it is still a popular idea for those trying to prevent aging. Given the known benefits of the metabolism of this diet, it is no wonder that people believe that regular fasting will help them stay alive and healthy.

As you can see, there are many benefits to following a fast-food diet. We have only touched on a few of them, but there have been many studies on the effects of this diet and why it may be useful for you. If you are trying to improve your mental health, live longer, lose weight, or gain more energy, indirect fasting can improve your life.

Issues Associated with Being Overweight

The kidneys work to clean the blood, removing impurities and water through the urine. It helps regulate blood pressure, which keeps the body healthy and active. When the kidneys are injured, and they cannot filter the blood as it is called kidney disease. When the filter is not right, the waste can build up in the body. Too much fat increases blood pressure and diabetes which is one of the major causes of kidney disease. According to recent studies, even when the condition is not present, obesity can directly cause kidney disease, especially if uncontrolled.

Diseases of Behavior

Steatohepatitis (non-alcoholic steatohepatitis (NASH)) also called fatty liver disease, occurs due to fat formation in the liver, which causes damage. This fatty liver can cause a number of injuries including liver failure, cirrhosis (tumor tissue), severe liver damage, etc. Occasionally, fatty liver disease may not permit the symptoms of an illness such as hepatitis B but not as a result of excessive drinking.

Osteoarthritis

Osteoarthritis is a health problem that causes pain and stiffness in the joints. This health issue is always related to age and injury. It usually affects the bones in the lower back, the waist, the knees, and the hands. Obesity is one of the common risk factors for developing osteoarthritis. Other factors include heredity, aging, and injury.

More pressure is put on the joints due to the extra weight. The bones and joints covered in fibrous tissue become tired due to the pressure of the fat and body weight. Also, high body fat can mean dangerous substances in the blood that may increase the risk of inflammation.

Sleep Apnea

One or more shortness of breath produces this problem when you are asleep. People with this condition can have heart failure, focusing on difficulty and daytime sleepiness. According to research, sleep deprivation can be caused by obesity. This is because a person with a lot of fat around their neck may have fewer airways. In fact, small airways can cause difficulty in breathing, or breathing can be very loud, often referred to as shortness of breath. In chronic cases, breathing can stop for a while before it can continue. Also, fat stored in the neck can increase the risk of inflammation caused by sleep apnea.

Stroke

When the flow of blood to the brain stops, there are high chances of experiencing a stroke. When this happens, it means that one may get ischemic stroke because of the blockage of the blood that flows to the brain. Sometimes one may experience another type of stroke called Hemorrhagic, which happens due to the rapturing of blood vessels. When blood pressure increases because of obesity or obesity, stabbing is more likely. Other problems commonly associated with strokes include heart disease, high blood sugar, and high cholesterol.

Understanding Your Body and Intermittent Fasting

Before you begin with any periodic fasting program, you need to fully understand your plan and know if it will go down well with your body type or not. Adjusting your portions or how often you eat may work better than occasional fasting. No two people will respond to a set of incentives in the same way. So you choose the one that works best for you.

Want to give it a shot? Then dip your toe in the water to feel it. Go all day fasting without eating a bite. There is no problem. You will feel very uncomfortable, and you will have a lot of empathy. At this point, you will want to throw in the towel and leave. Your productivity may decrease, headaches, and other symptoms may begin within a few hours after remembering to eat. If you are strong enough to handle this and decide to go ahead with the program, where do you set up your tent? Just go through the types of fasting listed and figure out which one works best for you. You should also know that fasting can be done permanently or stopped when the desired weight is obtained. To keep in touch with how much weight you have lost, keep track of your calorie intake, fasting times, and your weight for longer.

Cleaning System

You can always come up with your own fasting program with ay features included in other fasting programs. To do this, however, make sure you are not new to the whole process. To build your plan, here are a few tips to have in the back of your mind.

- All programs have features called mealtimes and fasting times.
- The time you eat is much shorter than the last time.
- Make sure you do not go into starvation mode, which starts about 38 hours of food insecurity. The maximum allowable fasting time is 24 hours. Anything after this contradicts itself.

The Journey to Having a Successful Fasting Program Can Be Very Difficult.

Here are some guidelines to help you get through the field.

- Take it one step at a time to understand what the program covers. Try a little fasting program. You don't want to jump first into something he or she may have been doing for you. You can start fasting once every three weeks before slowly reducing the time frame as you wish.

- Not one system works the same way for everyone. So choose a plan and use it for your taste.

- You will need to be fully aware of how your body responds to a periodic fasting program. Your body plan will determine what you eat, what time to eat, when to exercise, how many calories, etc. Putting all these things together will ensure that you are in control of the fasting process and, ultimately your weight.

- You don't want to hurry when you see fat flying through your bones. Many of us are impatient and get rid of certain foods one after the other because they don't work fast enough. You need to understand that for health purposes, losing weight should be a slow and slow process. Losing two pounds a week is just okay.

- Take part in your daily activities while you are in a hurry as this is a time-travel method. Being inactive will keep your mind focused on food, and you can guess the result here.

The most important piece of advice is that you do not have to eat all the time. As with health, there is a time for everything we have set for ourselves. So it also applies to your diet. Fasting is not ironclad, work on it, and set up a plan that works for you.

Chapter 5: Successful, Fasting, Eating and Eating

Most people will experience the effect of periodic fasting. They eat well in certain windows and make sure food is healthy when eaten. However, if you want to improve your performance and burn more fat, it is important to add your workout to your daily routine. This chapter outlines the proper training and exercise strategies to take during a quick workout.

In fact, a recent study by the Swedish Institute of Sports and Health Science showed that lowering the total amount of carbohydrates in a diet can cause the body to burn calories more efficiently and increase the capacity for muscle growth. In this study, ten cyclists who received an hour of interval training reached 64% of their maximum aerobic capacity. Glycogen levels are low or normal in their diet or before exercise intervention.

Ten biopsies were performed before the exercise and three hours after the exercise. The results indicate that exercise in glycogen depletion can increase mitochondrial biogenesis. This is the process by which new mitochondria can form within the cell. The authors of this study believe that low glycogen intake may be helpful in improving the oxidative capacity.

Part of the reason for making your current fasting state is that the body has ways to protect and protect your tissues from debris. So, if you naturally use very little energy during fasting, the body will start to break down other tissues, but it will not slow down the active tissue you are using.

Exercise While Maintaining Muscle Mass

Many experts believe that about 80% of the health benefits from a healthy diet come from food. The rest will be from sports. This means that if you want to lose more weight, you need to focus on eating the right foods. However, it is important to note that exercise and diet are necessary.

Investigators learned the details of the 11 participants who participated in the "Big Loser" program. Total body fat for participants, total energy cost, and resting rate were measured three times. At the beginning of the program, the measurement was taken after six weeks and 30 weeks. Using a personalized food model, researchers can calculate the effects of diet and exercise changes on weight loss to understand how everyone achieves this goal.

Researchers have found that diet itself is a major cause of weight loss. However, about 65% of the loss of weight originates from body fat. It happens due to the leaning of muscles. Exercise alone will result in a decrease in fat and a slight increase in the number of soft muscles.

Exercise and Fasting Together

If you want to find a workout program that works out, add high-intensity training, and occasional fasting, you need to combine certain things. When you do this, if you feel that you do not have enough energy to keep up with exercise, it's time to make some changes. Often reducing hours in an empty stomach will make the difference. Fasting indoors can make you feel good. If you can't hurry, it's time to change your strategy.

There are two important points to keep in mind when exercising at regular intervals. The first is about mealtimes. Fasting indoors is not just about limiting calories. You don't have to starve yourself to get the best results. Instead, this is just time to plan meals, so you don't have to eat most of the day. You can eat out of a small window, maybe at night or later in the day. So, if your dinner is limited to between 4 and 7, you will be fasting for 21 hours.

For most people, it is good to fast for 12 to 18 hours. Most people like to fast for 16 hours because it fits their busy schedule. You can find a way that best suits your needs while making sure you get all the benefits.

If you can't completely stop eating during the day, you can limit your dose of small, simple hypoglycemic foods. This includes cooking a pack of boiled eggs, Whey protein, vegetables, and fruits every four to six hours. It doesn't matter what you decide to eat; it is best to avoid eating at least three hours before bedtime. Doing this can help you minimize the damage to your system and can make periodic fasting easier.

In addition, on the day of exercise, you should break the fast by restoring food. On days when you have to exercise while fasting, you need to take a snack of about 30 minutes after your workout. Adding Whey Protein made to a meal can help rejuvenate the body's tissues.

After dinner, it's best to fast and have a great dinner that night. Eat a balanced diet after each workout. This will ensure that your body receives the demand for energy, and no muscle or brain damage. Don't skip these foods and make sure you get them within 30 minutes of your use.

If you think it is difficult to fast for 12 to 18 hours, you can get the same benefits from exercise and fasting by eating breakfast and exercise as soon as you have an empty stomach in the morning. This is because eating a large meal before exercise, especially foods with high carbohydrate content, will hinder the sympathetic nervous system and reduce the effect of fat burning during exercise.

So many people are taught that they need to get more carbohydrates before exercise in order to gain endurance and see results; it goes against your goal. Eating carbohydrates activates the parasympathetic nervous system, which promotes energy storage and stores calories and carbohydrates in the body. If you are exercising and doing quick exercises from time to time, this may be the last thing you want, so it is better to exercise faster to get better results.

Use Your Fitness Tips a Lot

Exercise is not necessarily difficult. Exercise and lots of exercise can help you feel good, build muscle, and lose weight. Other ways to ensure that you do well during regular exercise include:

- Start small - if you've never done a weight-lifting plan before, you need to start slowly. Even if you return to an existing workout, it's important to remember the changes and slow down until you know how they will affect your performance.

- Increase your weight when you feel relaxed - it's important to continue to gain weight when you start to feel comfortable. As time goes by, the weight used to start the work will start to feel easier, and if you don't make any changes, you will find that the results will be slower. This does not mean that you want to force your body to exceed the limit, but rather that if you want to achieve continued success; you need to increase the difficulty of a regular exercise program.

Reduce the Number of Times and Gain Weight Is Best for Soft Muscles - If at All

If you want to build muscle, consider reducing the amount of repetition when you increase your weight. This will get rid of your body faster and give you better results.

Don't forget to warm up and relax - just because you have to change your eating habits and can't give you excuses to slow down the warmth and calm of your daily workout. It takes at least five minutes to stretch the muscles at the beginning and end of the operation, which not only improves athletic performance but also reduces the chances of injury.

Focus on bodybuilding - sometimes paying too much attention to the weight it can lift while exercising. However, having the right form is really important. It is better to exercise properly and lightweight than to gain weight and not do it right.

Chapter 6: Intermittent Fasting Diet.

In the whole chapter, we will look at fat storage inside our bodies and how to burn it.

How This Fat Is Stored and Burnt?

This type of fasting has been looked at as a helpful factor to consider in one's health as it burns fats and eventually makes one lose his weight. How is this tool effective? Before we go in detail on this issue you are supposed to know how your body stores energy it acquires from intakes, how it uses the energy, and the roles played by body hormones in the body functions. In the circle of human life its either you store energy in your body or burn that energy and calories attained by body tissues every day.

This concludes that your body is either using energy (sugar) or storing it inform of fat or glycogen. Whether you are mobile or immobile in your daily chores you have the ability to burn your fats and calories and even sugar that is stored in excess amounts in the body.

According to statistics, mobility does not play many roles in the fat burn process; researchers suggest a 2:3 percentage in the loss equation. Human beings burn fat in many ways even when they are not moving, they will still lose it upon a smart guide discussed in the below chapters. The body of a human being will tend to expend its energy as it does its normal functioning according to BMR and BMR.

Even though the body might be consuming and burning all the calories all the excess is stored for use, and it's the energy stored that makes intermittent fasting a successful deal. As much as your body stores sugar and burns it weight loss is geared by less eating, and more exercises will this book will be your first beat of gearing success in losing weight and maintaining your body healthier. You will see the results at the end, and count fails to get back to normal eating and lifestyle.

What should you do to make it a success in losing weight? To get the image of all these two principals will not only guide you but also be of a great impact if practiced with concern; the principle of storing and burning sugar and how that sugar can be used for energy is your first option. The second principle is the role played by body hormones in the body functions.

How Is Energy Stored in Our Bodies?

The body of a human body can store energy in two ways, either in fat or glycogen. For instance, if you take a yum diet it is broken down into small and simple macronutrients ready to be absorbed in the body bloodstreams and transported in the body tissues for normal body functioning. In these processes, carbohydrates are broken down into glucose that is transmitted in the body cells for energy and with the excess stored as Glycogen through the glycogenesis process. Our bodies are meant for storing energy as fats, which are eventually broken down into energy through a process known as lipolysis, but only when it is in huge amounts is when is stored.

How Is the Stored Energy Used in Body Functioning?

Immediately the body cells require a lot of energy than the one needed (low blood sugar) by the bloodstreams. Glycogen is converted to glucose by the glycogenolysis process. The glycogen stores fats and then get back it after being emptied to digest the available fats by lipolysis process raising blood sugar level to its normality, and the whole process will mean breaking down of fats. To summarize on the process;

•	Excess glucose is turned to glycogen and stored once it is activated by a high

sugar level.

•	 Once glycogen is filled up the glucose stored in excess is converted to fat and

stored.

•	Blood sugar level drop symbolizes glycogen breakdown to glucose

•	Fat is broken down once the glycogen stores are emptied

To this far we have roughly looked on how our bodies function through storing of fats, breaking them down into energy/burning them. Below we will discuss the hormones responsible for controlling these processes.

Hormones

Body hormones are the most associated with one's moods. They play a big role in someone's weight loss. The secretion of hormones is of a great deal with your body as it rises from glands, each with a purpose. For instance, when blood sugar level rises, it plays the role of releasing insulin. Below are the key hormones responsible for weight loss.

Insulin Rising of blood sugar level activates insulin release leading to low blood sugar. This is because insulin helps in the transmission of glucose in the body cells for energy with the excess insulin taken into the liver. This makes the insulin to operate with much ease and start breaking down fats into glycogen. When you eat, your blood sugar level rises to stimulate the production of insulin that is of great importance. High secretion of insulin is activated by huge intakes of carbohydrates and lots of eating which results in the constant intake of sugar in the body. Since the main role of insulin is to store energy constant intake and eating of carbohydrates means that your body is storing a lot of carbohydrates which means that failure to take action to burn it will lead to weight gain and you will be at the risk of getting back to the weight loss procedures.

This is because the insulin will begin to resist its functions and the body will have to resist its functioning which means that more secretion of insulin will have to take place to fight against high sugar levels in the blood which will lead to overload of storing forcing liver to make convert of fats into glucose and start gaining weight through fattening. This is because glucagon is broken down once blood sugar level drops in order to raise blood sugar in the bloodstreams. Glucagon also stimulates adipose tissues that break the fat stores for bloodstreams. You are supposed to know that glucagon does the opposite of insulin in support of body functions. This leads to an energy-burning state which is geared by when insulin releases two hormones, which will be discussed in the chapters below.

Human Growth Hormone (HGM)

The weight loss perspective you need to know is that Human growth Hormones are triggered by enough sleep, low blood sugar level, and enough exercising. Human growth hormone functioning depends on different factors; for example, when children are sleeping their HGM will help their bones to grow but to the same as for adults. In relation to weight loss, the human growth hormone helps to regulate low blood sugar by breaking down the stored fats and growing muscles. Once you are an underweight loss, you are needed to lean on the activity of HGM and its production in your body.

Under endocrinology, the human brain senses insulin-like growth factors in the body and suppresses HGM release in the body and this clarifies the method of diagnosing overproduction of HGH which is done by giving sugary drink to the affected hence promoting drop of the HGH level drop with the meaning that high consumption of carbohydrates and sugary foods will not only go to give you high blood sugar but also overturn the release of HGH. These hormones do not stimulate adipose tissue break down to store fats, which means that it is never in the system with the role of stimulating muscle growth and bone density. This is caused by the release of fat cells, which means that the more fat cells you are having, the more leptin is released in the body to help in stabilizing weight by regulating hunger, appetite, and satiety.

Leptin

Leptin level refers to the number of fats you are having with your body. The more body fat you have, the more leptin you are having in your bloodstreams. The less body fat you are having, the less leptin your bloodstreams will be having, with the aim of losing weight drop-in body fat that leads to a drop-in leptin level resulting in an increase in appetite. With this mechanism in your tips, you will understand the reason why the loss of weight makes someone feel like he/she eat a whole horse if allowed to. Just Like insulin, the body can develop leptin resistance because when you are overweight, the excess amounts of leptin in the bloodstreams might make the body to build immunity, meaning that even when you carry a lot of fats, the leptin doesn't work well to overwhelm your appetite, which may encourage overeating and cause inequality of the hormones discussed above.

Eating on the intermittent fast is very simple and with very many complications as it is always upon your choice to continue with your eating behaviors or add a new diet and eventually see the end results. The ketogenic diet can better you if allowed to as it helps in limiting your carbs and reducing hunger and eventually burn your fats quickly. While under intermittent fasting there is no need to go on a specific meal as you can rarely get results at the end, in fact, you are supposed to eat healthy food on this diet plan since with this diet plan one is expected to drop his eating habit during the day to not more than eight hours but note that using these time gaps to eat fast foods such as snacks will still drive you into issues for you will not be able to lose your weight once you eat these fast foods as they are rich sources of calories with some other unhealthy foods which will give you a huge intake in every time you have them as food.

Though you might have small intakes of these unhealthy foods, you will stop your entire process of burning fats and fail to increase your weight loss effort. To this far you might have noticed that eating snacks and fast foods will definitely fail your effort of weight loss because they are unhealthy and causes the same problems that you encounter before starting the process.

When you have an unhealthy diet, you will find that you are hungry often and you will struggle with getting through your fasting periods with less comfort because many processed and fast foods contain chemicals and preservatives that are designed to make you hungry often in the event where you intend to start prayer and fasting even if for a whole month it's the high time to start eating healthier food or diets. This does not mean that you are supposed to avoid junk foods and sweets on occasions as it does not have set guidelines for what you are allowed to eat as it simply sets the times that you are allowed to eat. Eating a little snack and junk meal is fine. As long as you have it during your eating windows and only do it on occasions though it may be hard, always eating healthier will provide you with better results.

The trick to making this practice successful is always eating healthier. The first thing that you need to put into consideration is eating plenty of fruits and vegetables or including them in every diet with much majoring on fresh produces as they are best because they provide lots of essential nutrients that your body requires to stay healthy. Consider filing your plate with fruits and vegetables in every meal so that you ensure that you are getting the nutrients that are essential for someone's health. Eating a wide variety of products is very important to ensure that you are getting what your body requires without adding in lots of calories.

Next, you are supposed to go with some good sources of protein. You should consider options like lean ground beef, turkey, and chicken. Having some bacon and other fatty meats on occasion is acceptable, but don't overdo it. Eating a lot of fish will help you get the healthy fatty acids that the body needs to function appropriately.

Healthy sources of dairy help someone to stay lean while giving his body the calcium it needs. You can have some options like milk, yogurt, cheese, sour cream, and many others. Make sure that you monitor the salts and sugars that are not healthy for your body.

You are accepted to have some carbs on such a diet. Carbs have become a bit of a bad reputation because very many diet plans recommend that you avoid them. The most important thing is eating the carbs that are healthy and of benefit to your health. Foods such as snacks, White bread, and pasta are sugar made in disguise and should be avoided. Going with both whole grain and whole wheat options when it comes to your carbs will ensure that you get all the nutrition that you will need.

Taking a well-balanced meal will be the key to ensuring that you feel good when you are on an intermittent fast as your body will remain strong as well as healthy at all times. You will be able to mix the meals that you choose, so as to get the best results when you go on this kind of fasting.

You can also have with you a snack and remember how often you are having it because when you are eating junk foods, you will get disappointed when you go to measure your weight to the scale as you will find that you are adding your weight instead of losing it. You can have as many pleasures on occasions as well as many junk meals, but make sure that it is not exceeded in your diets.

Using the Ketogenic Diet with Intermittent Fasting

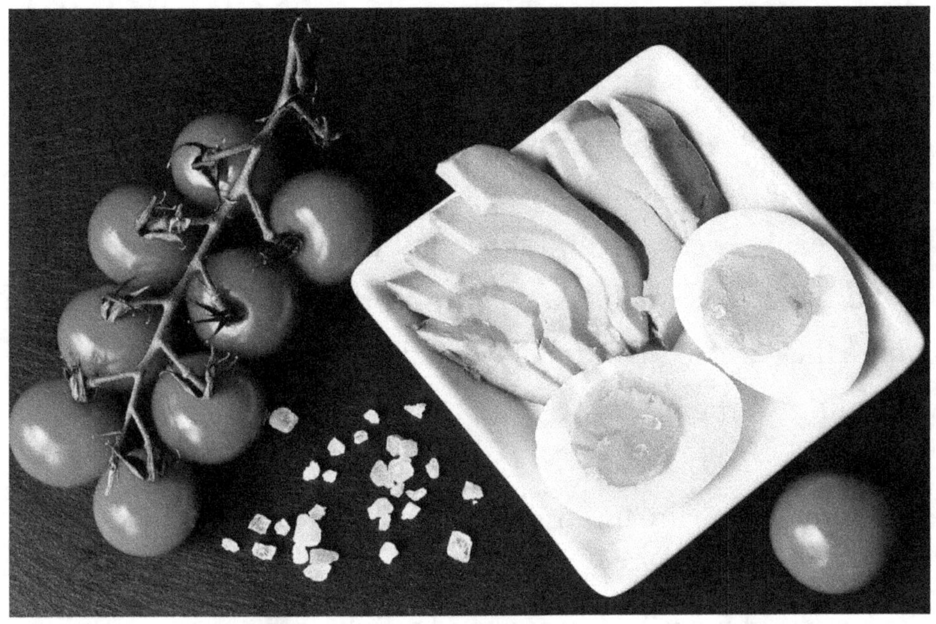

Many people choose to go for a ketogenic diet while doing an intermittent fast to help them remain healthy. The ketogenic diet includes high fat, moderate proteins, and low carb diets that help someone to burn fat quickly while reducing his dependency on sugary meals. There is a lot to love with this diet plan because when combined with the intermittent fasting, someone is sure to get great results in no time.

It's possible to use both of these diet plans together. Intermittent fasting is focused on the times of day when you will eat, and the ketogenic diet on what to eat during those periods.

For someone who would like to balance his blood sugar level and want to lose weight more efficiently, combining these two diet plans together will be very effective.

 For intermittent fasting, you should limit the hours that you can eat. Instead of spreading your meals and snacks throughout the day, you should limit it to just a few hours. Most people choose to only eat between ten and six and fit their macronutrients into that time. Others will take two or three days during the week where they are not allowed to eat and fit their nutrients into the other days of the week.

The point is, you are limiting the amount of time that you eat, forcing you to think about the foods you consume. You also get the benefit of more fat burning and weight loss, when practicing intermittent fasting.

During the times when you are allowed to eat, you will need to stick to the macronutrients that we have learned above that are approved for the ketogenic diet. You will still remain with high fat and moderate protein plan even while on intermittent fasting. You will be required to be more cautious about the times you eat the major nutrients though you can still follow the ketogenic diet plan.

If you want to get these benefits of intermittent fasting or you want to increase your weight loss efforts, then adding this diet in with the ketogenic diet is the most effective. You can test with different types of intermittent fasting options that are available and see which one fits into your schedule for the best of you. Of course, if you find the ketogenic diet effective or intermittent fasting very difficult, you can at all times stick with the ketogenic diet and not fast and still see good results.

It is very vital to recall that you don't have to follow the ketogenic diet plan if you are on an intermittent fast. Many people go choose other healthy diets instead of choosing to go on the ketogenic diet. Though, there are many people who will choose to go with the ketogenic diet along with intermittent fasting because it is very easy to follow, and it allows one to lose more fat.

Eating on the intermittent fast does not have to be difficult for you. You can opt to pick out the foods that you want to eat, although it is important to go with food that is fresh and whole, and that will fill you to burn your fat and help you see yourself losing weight.

Chapter 7: Tips to Help You Succeed in Intermittent Fasting

In order to ponder the number of intervals to fast, it will be more viable if one has to choose a style that befits him well. There are different approaches to follow. It could be 12:7 method, or 10:4. The first one is fasting for twelve hours that is, through the better part of the day (even during the sleeping hours), then eight hours to eat food. Then 10:4 methods it entails ten-hour fast followed by a four-hour eating window. Both of these provisions a person can opt to choose when to start even as one pleases. You can cease your fast at noon and consume food at seven in the evening.

Moreover, if the breakfast is more important to you, you can opt to partake late-day snacks then eleven to six evening window to which could prove better for you. Another person could prefer a long span of fasting. This could be composed of 4:2 approaches; this constitutes consuming food for four days in a week and taking the two days as fasting days. The amazing thing about this dieting is that it be customized for someone to choose what he finds appealing or get the same sort of results.

Some of these alternatives could be: having easy swaps of options will make one not run out of order cooks. The positive side of intermittent fasting is its simplicity. Do not resort to unnecessary ways of cooking your own food from the rest of the family meals. For instance, one can make a dish of pasta mixed with Bolognese stew for an evening meal, or spaghetti noodles, for the group and stewed noodles for him. Or offer a plate of lukewarm tortillas and heartwarming lettuce for wraps. These sorts of swaps can take a very small amount of time to prepare. There will be times when interval fasting will be daunting to adapt because someone will have to change some dieting patterns, but the efficacy can come in many ways. Then, in the long run, it can be easier to enhance your energy, lose weight gains, curb against diabetic maladies, cancer, and junk foods.

The intermittent fasting is best than other alternatives out there, but it needs a lot of effort. Some of the things one can bear in mind are: gulping a lot of water which can make one hydrated, and belly become a bit fuller; otherwise, the stomach will always be tormenting due to hunger pangs. Drinking tea and coffee will suppress hunger and unwanted appetites. But do not take caffeinated drinks when about to sleep because that will make one unable to doze. Make your mode of life to be hectic, the reason being that on an empty stomach one can be less active. If you are busy you can attain a lot, avoid hunger, and avoid long periods of hunger spells that appear like long periods of years. Please do not be hard on yourself. When it comes to new eating habits you can make your days filled with many activities. You should be flexible because intermittent fasting comes with its downsides. You do not have to go with the crowd. Mixing and matching the schedule that works is good. Remember, intermittent fasting is about having the self-will to do as one pleases.

Then a person could try to make it a monthly trial. Meaning the probationary period could be from three weeks to four weeks. If someone is not adapting well, it means that there is not ample time to make adjustments. So a certain amount of time is needed to check out whether it works or not. Additionally, one can opt to experiment with alternative fasting methods. What could be feasible to a particular person might be not workable to another person. If you discern that one type of fasting ids better and more applicable than the other application that fits you. The point is that the experiment is all that is needed to make a solid conclusion. Then a person can commence by delaying and denying himself breakfast drastically. Pushing a breakfast in a gradual process every week or so, then you can come into terms with intermittent fasting without too much ado.

For example, if you usually take food at nine o'clock morning you can wait up till ten o'clock and then consume your week's breakfast. Then you can move on taking the same breakfast to ten o'clock. Then you can continue shifting the eating patterns up to midday.

During the start of morning hours, taking a few cupsful of water will be okay. Remember that the reason you feel so hungry in the morning hints that you took nothing as food. So the first thing is to get a glass of water as someone wakes up. Then if there is a need for gaining weight and toning up, it makes sense to it would be wise to resort to weight exercises as a routine. While it will not be wise to start too many things, especially when someone is on a startup route, but as soon as the body adapts to the fasting style, there is a need to move things up. Then there will always be surprises because the body can sustain itself despite too much intensity and many hindrances along the path of improvement.

Intermittent fasting every person has to live up at a time. It can be fascinating as long as there is a balance in the long run.

The typical diet is all about the 'forbidden foods,' but the intermittent fasting means that you cannot preplan your meals. Meaning there is no way to turn around the hours, so long as there is no constancy. Consequently, there is no way someone cannot involve himself, as far as a delicious and a fake dessert does not end up into nine to eight.

Recall being around all nice smelling foods; there is a heavy temptation to get a bite. So make it a policy to get out of the house. If you have kids who needed your attention, exert yourself in an activity that keeps your mindset occupied?

There is a need to take more protein foods and healthy fats because sufficient protein in every meal makes an individual have a controllable appetite and aid in buttressing muscles with energy.

An excellent amount of fats to more energy and a long span of a full belly. We can give credit to many dieticians for giving us many advises on our meals, but sometimes we need to try best to check what works for us or not. The majority of people consume too many carbohydrates and take other unbalanced portions. But the problems can be rectified by taking into consideration the macros of the foods we take. Additionally, when you are taking your favorite delicacy make it a deal that you fill your plate to the brim so that the next window would be easy as possible.

Avoid the worst of all junk foods most of the times people can resort to non-bodybuilding foods but always make it a resolve to have a balanced diet so that you provide your body with sufficient nutrition even if you are about to fast.so it is essential to note that a huge part of intermittent fasting is to gain the amount calories which has been snapped up during the eventual part of the week-long fasting.

If you drench up your body with high– calorie junk when you are embarking on an eating window what could be the consequence is, your hard work is being undone. Recall making decisive options entirely will finally enhance the overall effectiveness of your weight harm efforts, assured.

This journal could prove to be gigantic and important because it can make you keep track of everything from the outset. Someone can use modern gadgets if there he finds that more viable, but some old-fashioned folks using a journal proves easier.

Ideally, it can help also to count the number of no-fasting hours, mood swings at that moment, both positive and negative. This way you can monitor the progress. If there are fits of anger let us say on Tuesday the reason could be that the body is coming into grips with the new fasting you have been up to or that a certain diner you took is still being channeled to your system.it is so hard to discern if there are patterns of loss gains, or moving on the right track healthy lifestyle if you do not document. The best thing is to take a picture of oneself or look yourself in a mirror so as to have something to meditate on later or maybe survey progress

Ride out the Hunger Waves

Pangs of hunger do not endure for a long time, but they can be harrowing. But the moment they emerge, they can be intolerable so you can resort to huger waves. Opposite of the popular opinion that when hunger comes up, it eats up you inside more and more till you sense death, but it subsides depending on the way you can make it through. When someone is hungry what happens to their body is hydration. a particular body may exhibit dehydration by having symptoms of hunger when what needs to be done is just take a cup of water.

Start Gradually

When embarking on a new lifestyle or grappling with intermittent fasting the food advice is to do it gradually. Everybody needs time to adapt and transition itself without haste. For instance, if you are fasting through the normal dinner time until six in the morning make sure you see yourself through without any food around even the ensuing day even stretching up to lunchtime. Some folks have the inclination to get into anything new without any forethought, and they push themselves through the hard spans of times and cravings. But the best of all conveniences gradual process is the best way to travel no matter how rocky it is. In conclusion, we can draw a lot from intermittent fasting; also, we should not have unfounded expectations from weight loss, good body posture no matter how strict the fasting path might be.

Meanwhile, there will be jiffies of weight loss, as the body's systems funnel itself to the trials. But everything will most likely totally change eventually after the fasting period. This can be visible during the initial weeks of transition as the body will be trying cling on to everything that to the time it figures itself out. But the time it figures the process, later on, everything will come to join the dotted path to follow through. Every diet is meant to have weight gains or loss paradigm. This could be part of weight gain or loss, and it cannot be controlled. But there are consistent and feasible measures that will prove adaptable and workable, but the futile thing is to try to change things up whimsically because this can spiral into a more problematic conundrum of events. Whereas if you pursue a positive course and exert oneself to the good work, the fine results will be eminent and visible before you come to realize.

Always bear in mind any strenuous physical activity requires precautions in the same case our intermittent fasting needs lot care because our very souls are involved and depend on it. The health benefits cannot be underestimated because it can prevent diseases and enhance spiritual wellbeing. Even those who are overweight can help to cut down the body mass as well. There are those with eating disorders, so they should not strenuously exert themselves on it. So in hindsight, timing your meals can improve your wellbeing, control weight, and most of all, make you physically active. So the resolve to achieve better results is good regardless of distractions one has to encounter along the way, but the payback will be worth pursuing.

Chapter 8: Most FAQ(s) on Intermitted Fasting

There are simple questions that need to arise from your mind about intermittent fasting. We will be discussing these questions very clearly. What is it needed for intermittent fasting is to enjoy the best out of it to be a simple practice and be of help to you?

Who Should Fast and Not?

This type of fasting is meant for everyone who wishes to reduce his/her fat and the willingness to make it a success in losing weight. As we discussed earlier, it is meant for reducing calories by paving a focus on healthy eating. This reflects that you are not supposed to get into this plan if you need special nutrients in your body due to its characteristic of less food consumption. For instance, if you are pregnant, breastfeeding, and underweight, this diet plan should not concern you at all; otherwise, you should ask for a recommendation from your doctor.

Group two type of people who should not attempt this diet plan are those suffering from Diabetes either type 1 or type 2 and high uric acid they are supposed to take the caution of seeking doctors' advice.

Can Someone Starve While Fasting?

It is a misconception that you can starve while fasting as long as you are healthy fit as intermitted fasting is an effective tool in reducing fats stored in the body and burning them for energy during the starving days. When it comes to fasting, it is all about your wellness, some opinions posted by people against fasting myths are that fasting makes one starve, lose muscles, feel hungry and start overeating after undergoing fasting. As we discussed earlier this is false as all these myths make one lose weight, burn fats, and overcome unnecessary fatness. For instance, if you are struggling with being overweight this is the right book for your weight loss. The myth of starving, which is the most common, is greatly reasoned out by the eating that someone does in a whole year and the intake of calories in those diets with losing one whole week without food. No starving that can be evident in this fasting its benefit and benefit. Just try it and thank yourself later! The body of a human being can stay for even two weeks without food, and you are seen walking very comfortably and without anybody noticing whether you are fasting.

What Side Effects Do They Come with Fasting?

Several effects will come after you are done with your fasting. The effects that someone encounters with this type of fasting are very manageable if you wish to start. After getting back to normal when you are done with burning the stored fats in the body. For example, lack of roughage in the body processes will cause constipation, and since you have gone without food for time this comes as the first side effect. To do away with it you just need some purges to help you in improving your discomfort. The problem of stomach babbling is solved by drinking salty water whereas the problem of headaches that comes often in the first days of fasting is done away by eating salts every morning. You might come across other side effects such as heartburn and dizziness, but after resuming to normal the same you never have the feels at all.

How to Manage the Hunger

The hunger experienced during this time should not worry you as it will pass as it comes. Researchers say that hunger come in waves just like moving water to avoid this hunger while fasting you are supposed to take a soft drink immediately, and you will have no instance of claiming hunger you can also opt to take a cup of tea or coffee and forget about the waves though it will be experienced I the first and second day of fasting. With the third and fourth days, it will be normal to continue the rest of the days you feel of extending your fast. You will manage this because the body has fats that are digested to be a form of energy in the whole fast. Once the hunger pain waves are gone within the second day with the other days it is very cheap and easy for managing the fast. It is very important to have in mind that this is very manageable though for beginners it's a big deal in the first two days due to the habit of the body getting food all through. There two types of fasting 16:8 and 5:2. Practicing either of them is a true indication that you are making yourself strong and even preparing for a life of comfort without obese and free mobility. To prepare for this make sure that you take a balanced meal with every meal as it will make your body to remain strong always and ready. To be in the ability to make this manageable, also you don't leave behind caffeine in your meals because it is a good way to reduce hunger pains when they come in waves. During this type of fast ensure that you keep yourself busy all through to put your mind on the focus of what you are aiming at. If you are already committed to an exercise plan, then you are supposed to ensure that you exercise with much commitment before you break your fats so that your body can get the fuel it needs to make the most of your efforts.

Can Fasting Burn Muscle?

This is a misconception that dwells in almost everyone who fears to fast. This is a myth because, during the fasting periods, the body breaks down the glycogen into glucose to be used for energy purposes, and after the glucose is all gone, the body increases the fat it's breaking down and uses that for energy. Excess amino acids, which build up in the system proteins, can also be used for energy. Fasting is a practice that has been done effectively for a long time. It's safe and effective, and unless you go for weeks without eating there isn't a reason for worrying about losing excess muscles.

How do I break the fast? Once you are about to break the fast prepare a dish a minute before it is over. A pot of oatmeal is not a good choice; instead, choose an Omelet because it is healthy and has many nutrients. As the end of this fasting is not very nice as it puts one in the point of sustaining in the long moments.

Once you break your fast it is important to do away with moderation for multiple reasons. DO NOT OVER EAT!!! Eat a little dish to withstand a long period you stayed without food, do not also overwork until you resume to normal as the body tissues will have used the stored energy in the tissues.

Can Women Fast?

Women can fast with some exemption, such as if they are underweight, pregnant, or breastfeeding. This is because they require those extra nutrients and should not go so long without eating in intermittent fasting. Otherwise, it is perfect for women to fast as they have huge fats compared to men. Besides, the average weight loss with fasting is the same for men and women, and it is effective for both genders. Though starting intermittent fasting is a challenge for a beginner we are going to discuss tips that will enable you to fast effectively.

Drink a lot of water and prefer water rich in minerals and remain busy in your chores during fasting Drink coffee or tea as they are rich sources of caffeine to suppress your hunger
Find out a support group or a team to help you ride out the hunger waves
Try to go on a low-carb diet because it will help you to reduce your hunger and make your fasting as easy as possible.
Break a fast gently and avoid too much eating in the first days until you get used to normal.

Bonus Tips to Help in Maintaining the Proper Weight

Use of Spices

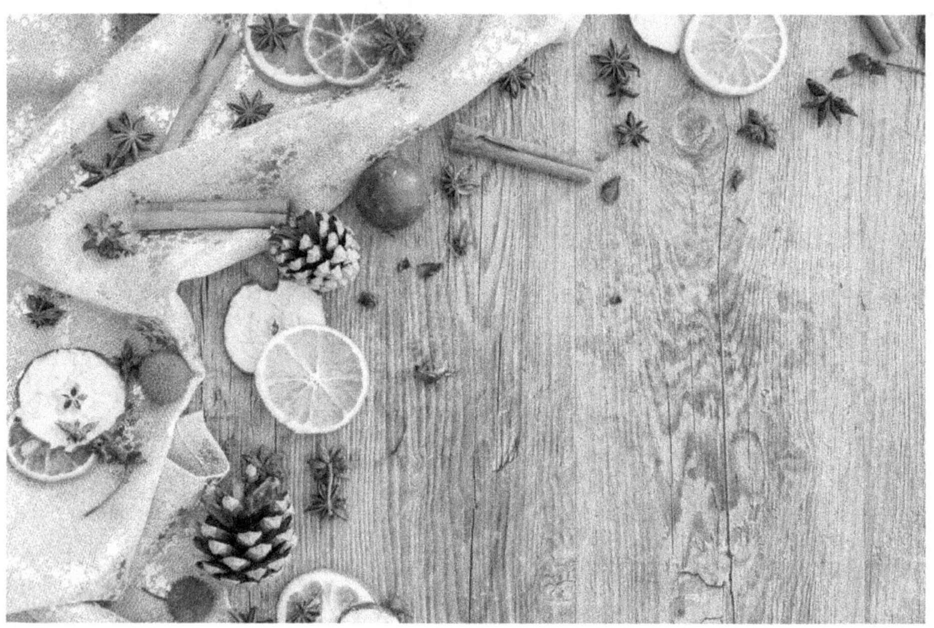

Spices have performed a number of functions ranging from flavor to medicinal purposes since the beginning of humankind. Archaeological studies have found spices from the ruins around the Nile District since 2800 BC. The various types of spices and herbs not only delight our scents, but they also work to preserve human bodies. Countries in the medieval period carried herbs and spices to great heights and used them for purposes ranging from funeral ceremonies, royal ceremonies, and treatments.

In these modern times, we have associated the spices most with the taste qualities they offer to our dishes. Going back to studying the ancient uses of these spices has begun to open a new vista to their potential as a coolant and protect against the powerful antioxidants of fat burning. According to one recent study, the American Journal of Clinical Nutrition reported that adding rich spices to polyphenol in a meat dish reduced the production of Malondialdehyde, which is a product of peroxidation of lipids and is thought to cause cancer. Other studies have confirmed the effectiveness of spices and herbs by using its antioxidant power to fight off harmful substances in our daily diet. For example, do you know that the meat and other products that you produce and like so contain carcinogens?

This, however, can be reduced to a minimum by the addition of spices that prevent the formation of computer-generated cancer. Heterocyclic amine complements are made up mainly of meat, poultry, and seafood that are cooked at high temperatures, especially over fire or frying. We can almost certainly avoid such an important part of our diet, so what do we need to do to reduce the risk associated with consuming such products? Just introduce spices and herbs to brighten up the flavor of your barbecue and products at the same time for you and your loved ones. Common ingredients such as cumin, turmeric, and dozens of others are helpful in reducing HCA production. Spices and herbs not only reduce your risk of cancer but also serve as a barrier and cure against many other diseases from diabetes to common colds.

A 2011 study revealed that cinnamon and cloves because of its high hypolipidemic properties reduced blood cholesterol by approximately 65% in subjects during the study period. How do you explain weight loss in a high-fat diet during reading? This is the effect of the spices added to the diet of the articles during the frame.

As you continue to experience the wonderful potential of herbs, it is important to increase your use of these anti-inflammatory drugs. You can combine the following steps along the way to good health;

Take herbs and herbs with standard health supplements and not for the extra benefit they can give you. It is appropriate to eat foods that are rich in antioxidants, e.g., Spices, herbs, vegetables, fresh fruits, etc. To make your meal a great experience. As long as studies are ongoing regarding a particular disease inhibition of spice skills, that should not stop you from taking antioxidant-rich foods. We know for sure that spices contain significant amounts of antioxidants, but the lack of information lies in how this relates to good health and the benefits it provides us that we use regularly.

Don't limit yourself to specific spice and herbs; check the entire rainbow light. By trying a little of this and adding some of that to your diet, you will be getting the best of the delicious and healthy ingredients they have.

You should take your spices and herbs in any way you can. If you find a garden, then it makes perfect sense that you can use many new spices. However, if you can get your hands on some new herbs, dried ones will do the job correctly and often and over new treatments. The UCLA School of Medicine's research into herbs and spices found that they keep their essentials even though they are dry.

Details of the specific health benefits can be substantially better compared to sugar, fat, and salt. Spices bring out the subtle flavor, aromas, and flavor of your dishes and are healthy for your body. If you are on a diet or are looking for ways to get rid of those stubborn body fats, spices can come in to replace sugar and other artificial particles. We are so attached to the traditional ways of satisfying our languages and not paying enough attention to our bodies that the most common spices available may not have been recognized. Cinnamon is a great place for sugar in your tea, coffee, cereals. Your taste buds may be at war with you at first, but gradually the taste you get becomes more normal as your body begins to experience the great health benefits associated with its use.

There are many ways that when combined can be of effective remedies to keep your health in good condition all the year. They are relatively cheap with the process of making them so simple that even a young child can put them together. So getting into the crust of the remedies, there are few spices that you can implement into your daily meal plans for a healthy life. With this, I will be putting out a few powerful spices that work with much ease and that you might take and mix with any menu you might choose to come up with.

As much as you take all these measures to be cautious, especially if you have any severe ailments and undergoing treatment with medications, you are supposed to get in touch with a general consultant before you consume any spice or herb.

Cinnamon

This is the spice that lowers someone's blood sugar because it possesses an aroma that is quite lovely. If you might be dealing with diabetes, either type 1 or type 2, this is one spice that should adorn in your kitchen cabinet all the time. This is because constant use of this spice gradually pulls you away from the grip of sugar, and makes your body to stop craving for the sweet things. The good thing with this spice is that you get great sweetness without the ability to have harmful effects due to lots of sugar in your system.

This can elevate your risks of coming down with complications associated with diabetes to avoid it add a sprinkle to your tea or coffee or a teaspoon to your juice or any of your favorite drink.

Ginger

This is a light-yellow rhizome that has a sharp and hot taste. It has anti-microbial and anti-inflammatory properties. The fat-burning qualities of ginger are supposed to be marveled at. It is considered to be a digestive fire that paves the way for someone's body to produce digestive enzymes that quickly breaks down nutrients. Moreover, it is an essential spice for the treatment of a lot of your everyday illnesses that you will typically take synthetic and potentially harmful substances into your body to cure. This spice takes care of body pains, common cold, aching of the joints, nausea, and a boatload of other sicknesses. Once taken regularly and on a daily basis either in the form of tea or incorporated into other meals, it serves as a very powerful agent in the reduction of high cholesterol levels in your body. This is a spice that costs someone next to nothing and is ideally suited for a lot of body types without any side effects that are associated with artificial chemical substances someone consumes.

It is one of the best ingredients in improving someone's poor digestion. To get your gastrointestinal system activated daily, you are supposed to ensure that you take a teaspoon of dried ginger powder with warm water and some honey and ensure that it is the first thing you do in the morn at least thirty minutes before having your breakfast. You may also take it in between meals during the day. You can choose to add ginger can to your meals in the fresh form to boil your beef and also sprinkle onto your food to give a boost in your digestion.

With this spice, it not only work on your internal organs but also serves the role of supplying the body's external needs with a soothing and efficient circulation of blood at the surface of the skin. For someone with sore muscles or joints, he/she can make a poultice by adding two teaspoons of dried ginger powder a cup of warm water and gently stir up until there is the formation of a fine paste. Apply it to the spot and massage it into your muscles and start enjoying a soothing relief. It is very relevant to ensure that this mixture does not come in contact with your nose or eye, and to perfect it you are required to ensure that you wash your hands properly after handling ginger because of its fiery nature.

Onion and Garlic

Both of these spices are excellent cholesterol-lowering abilities, but most folks stay away from them because of the pungent odor associated with them, especially garlic. They have been used for quite a long time for their medicinal properties and for spicing foods. Onion and garlic stimulate the production of digestive enzymes, which breaks down fatty acid deposits. Garlic has a broader spectrum of action compared to the onion, and its active ingredients are stronger than those found in onions. They are useful in the cleansing of the liver, lowering high blood pressure, bacterial infections and they are not limited to gastrointestinal disorders and the common cold.

So now let's get into the act of using these new spices effectively. You can start by grinding on cloves of garlic and onions by dicing them up and adding some vinegar and manage to make a zingy salad without forgetting a dash of honey that might add some much-needed mellow taste to the mixture. This is convenient in the treatment of respiratory tract problems. I expect that you know onions and garlic are used for cooking in boiling, steaming, or frying specific foods. The healing effect of these two great spices on our bodies cannot be over-estimated.

If you wish onions and garlic can be consumed in powder or oil forms this comes down to suit you at any given point of time. You may choose to dissolve the powder in warm water and drink or take a clove or two of garlic two to three times every day; all of this will depend on your choice. It is important to note that if you have issues with one's gallbladder, take a full berth around garlic and onions and keep walking once you taste them, you are going to have severe pains for quite a long time.

Turmeric

This plant has been referred to as the "Top Dog of Spices." It helps the breakdown of food down the system, purifies the liver, and getting rid of poisonous substances from the human body.

So there is no need to take an anti-inflammatory prescription that can have detrimental effects on you, but turmeric can go well with your body.

It can ease off stress, cure diabetic problems, remedy digestive problems, control the diabetic impacts, and the endless cases of diseases. It has an unmatchable capability to preserve foods. Due to its potential to prevent the virus, it has been verified to give a blow to cancer-causing pathogens. There are no documented cases of people being affected by the overconsumption of turmeric. Any person can take the ground form of turmeric with tea, or coffee even incorporating it with other meals. The importance of this kind of spice is that it breaks down the buildup of fats inside the tissues. The incessant use of turmeric can make and steer up the digestive system and the body's membrane be4coming glossy.

Those who have been taking ginger and turmeric, especially for a long time when they were craving alcohol as the addictive vice to them reported more mental tranquility and superficial improvement of overall confidence. Then a little wonder is that they sensed less craving to smoke and consume alcohol. Some other additional advantages of the same spices are minimized acne and other skin blemishes that ensue from sweating and hormones. The blistering creamy sparkle of this amazing spice gives someone an aura of mellowness to his coffee as breakfast. At the best of all times, this wonderful spice does not end any breakfast delicacy, but it is part and parcel of those who comprehend its usefulness. So in essence, everyone should be a darling of this first-rate spice and experience the advantages that stream out of it.

Cayenne Pepper

This is also a very piquant and hot spice. The very hotness results from the capsaicin which is ever-present in hot peppers from chili to jalapenos. Due to the existence of the active components in the peppers, you can get the identical paybacks from all of these spices. Its principal purpose is to give a new lease of life to our metabolism, almost double our normal functionality when we have any food devoid it. After a plateful of jalapeno spiced food like barbecue, pizza someone feels re-ignition of metabolism, and the heart pace becomes stabilized. This is a fulfilling way to limit your eating longings as you get jam-packed quickly while your metabolism upsurges at the same time. So this is one ordinate spice that can aid in the dropping of excess body weight in a fine way.

Chances are that we have some other fascinating recipes that can bring a smile to our hearts mostly when we wake up in the morning. The day becomes lightened – so trying up cayenne pepper and lemons is the best alternative. It gets you straight out of bed, lights up your day when you put it in your breakfast. So it is good to try cayenne pepper and squash of lemon. Simply squeeze the lemon juice into the jar or any apparatus and give it a sprinkle of the aforementioned pepper in it. It can provide a jolt of excellent feeling in your system.

Black Pepper

This an important herb for strengthening one's gastrointestinal glares, arousing appetite, and more so cleansing organs.
It also helps in more production of hydrochloric acid, which makes the digestive system more viable. It curtails common diseases like common cold, fevers, and allergens. There are some other acute ailments like anorexia, liver diseases, nervous breakdowns; all those can be cured by administering black pepper. As a fact just take two spoonsful of black pepper, lace-up it with some honey, and maintain that daily as healthy takings.

Cumin

Incredibly, this spice has been confirmed in many areas of study to burn Belly fats three times than any other confirmed methods. Mainly take a small amount of water or mix it with morning tea daily and keep surveillance of fats around the waist being erased out. This is just one incredible spice that has been showed in studies to burn belly fat three times faster healthier than any known method. Just a pinch of warm water or your tea two to three times daily and watch that spare tire around your waist deflate in no time.

Eating Spicy Foods

Tea of Different Flavors

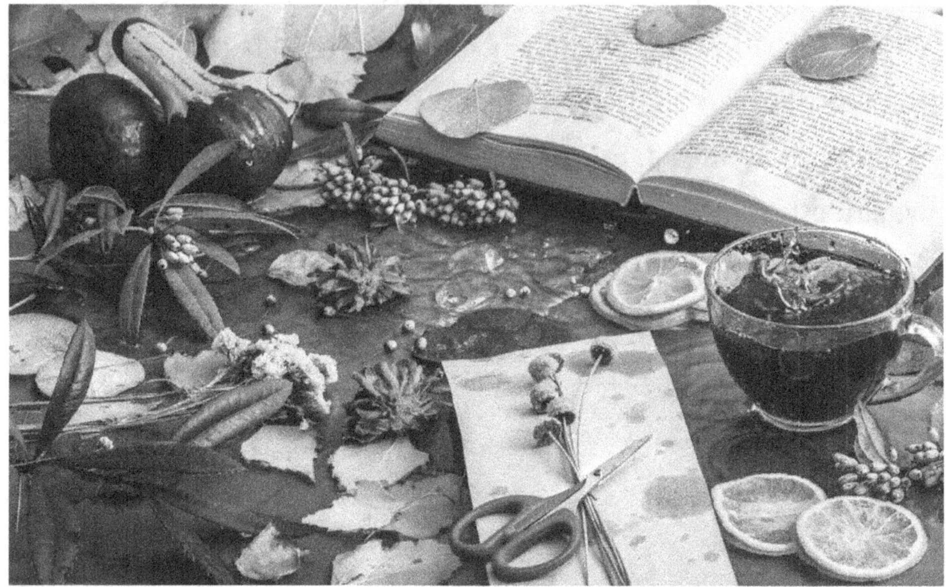

There is this health and vitality that a cup of well-prepared tea rich in antioxidants and earthy flavor can give your day. Entering into your comfort wander around in the evening with a book in hand or just be ready to break through that door to catch the train in the morning. Your cup of tea should give you the kind of comfort you won't get when your fingers are taken, and it should hold you back from accepting that you are not going anywhere else. Building your relationship with this beverage cup brings out some of the benefits of photo-free photography. A cup of tea can be as a standalone drink or eaten after a meal will help your food enter your stomach properly and help your digestion

I will give you a recipe for tea that you would love for life and pass it on to your kids. Now let's get into it. All you need for this recipe is some cinnamon, ginger, and honey. That's all. Surprised? Keep it simple and watch the magic as it unfolds in your body.

Find medium-sized ginger, wash, and peel it. Add it to the kettle and re-add one small cinnamon stick. Pour about 3 cups of water into the mixture and allow boiling for about 25 minutes. You can do more by increasing the number of ingredients if you have more tea lovers around you. You can also store in your refrigerator anytime you need a quick dose of life-giving elixir. So while this mixture is bubbling and the aroma from cinnamon stick fills every corner of your home, your body can't help but wait for the burning fluid that will bring much-needed relief from the forced fay.

After this mixture should boil for a few minutes, dip the liquid into the cavity. You can add honey if you need to soften it a bit, but it is not necessary since the cinnamon has a slightly sweet taste. The flavor explosion that mimics your taste buds is not the same thing you have ever had. It can be taken at any time of the day for your meals or alone.

Herbal Water

Do I need to continue the benefits that water has for life? I don't guess. However, drinking the recommended eight glasses of clean, dirty water can be a major challenge for many of us. Pure water is colorless, odorless, and tasteless. So how is it that we get around to just drinking "normal water" all day for the rest of our lives? We are merely enriching ourselves and stop living a tiring life. To start living a life full of fun with water to use with spices and spices. Get a mug and fill it with eight glasses of water, add three teaspoons of ginger to its wonderful digestive properties, and two slices of cucumber. Find the center lemon, close it, and place it in half. A few freshly squeezed mints leaves give a refreshing taste to the mix and also reduce your hunger pangs and reduce your sugar cravings.

Reduce Salt and Sugar Intake

Spices are great for giving us a taste of junk food and are important in helping us reduce the amount of sugar, salt, and other unwanted foods in our diet. Here are some of the easiest to follow tips for cutting out such food items.

To reduce the salt you use, use less spicy spices, e.g., ginger, onion, garlic, basil, curry, etc. It is also worth checking the labeled spices to make sure no sodium or some form of salt is added to the spice.

To keep your tongue happy, stick with "delicious" spices like cinnamon, nutmeg, allspice, Cardamom, etc. Gradually adding such spices to your daily drinks will see you become healthier as your tongue adapts to changes.

Rules to Consider

When cooking with spices or mustard, always make sure the recipe is well documented. However, when compiling a menu yourself, the amount and type of spice you add to any particular dish depends on your taste buds, and the occasion. Have you ever been in a jam about how to get a recipe that requires fresh spices and herbs but all you have is a dry compliment? Here's an easy way to get an equal amount of fresh spices

½ teaspoon dry ground herbs ¼ teaspoon dried herbs ¼ teaspoon freshly pulled

How many spices and herbs should you put in a bowl if you don't know how to do it? Follow these simple steps, and your diet will go well.

When cooking over a specified amount of people in a recipe, do not assume that it will double the amount of spices you should use. Increase the simple number of ingredients by ½ and taste it and decide when more is needed.

When hot peppers such as chili, jalapenos, cayenne, or red peppers are important ingredients in a bowl, add them slowly in small amounts because the taste becomes stronger as the cooking progresses.

Start any meal by adding ¼ of the necessary spices and adding it as slowly as possible.

The timing of adding spices to any meal is important, and it is also determined by the type of dish you prepare. When adding fresh spices meal, it will come to an end when your cooking is almost done because excessive heat can lead to a loss of flavor. Some very fragrant spices can be sprinkled with food just before it is served or as soon as the food leaves the fire. On the other hand, really heavy spices can last 10 to 15 minutes before a meal is finally ready.

Dried spices are best used in dishes that will be cooked for a long time, and emit their aroma slightly compared to fresh spices.
It is also important to keep your spices and herbs in order to maintain their quality for a very long time. To ensure you get the best out of your spices, store them in dark containers and perhaps on the shelves of your kitchen. Avoid areas where humidity and temperature can occur. Make sure you keep it in

air conditioners. When cooking, use dry spoons to take the quantity you need and do not pour your spices into the cooking pot to prevent the smoke from draining and ultimately damage your spices.

No matter how well you store your spice, like any food, it has a shelf life. So your used spices in powdered form, keep for 15 months and unrefined spices, for almost 30 months. To make sure that you do not eventually allow your spices to dissolve, buy small items first until you find out how long it takes to complete them.

Invalid Weight Loss Method

There is no doubt that there are many exercise programs and diet modes that allow you to achieve maximum weight loss with minimal effort, but it is certain that some of these techniques are ineffective, and even if they work, side effects can be harmful to your health. Therefore, you need to be very careful and consult your general practitioner before starting any weight loss program. You need to pay special attention to eating habits, especially when the weight is related to the disease. To avoid wasting time and money to solve things that might not ultimately work for you, here are some things that might not work for your weight loss, as well as suggested long-term alternatives.

Fat-Free and Sugar-Free

Regardless of the harmful effects of excess body fat, fat intake is not completely unhealthy. In fact, fat is one of the food nutrients necessary for the body to stay healthy. On the other hand, you may avoid avoiding sugar while avoiding exposure to fat, or avoiding fat that exposes you to more sugar. In fact, sugar-free products may contain artificial sweeteners, which will also help to gain weight. Even sugar-free drinks contain substances that enhance the taste, which in turn may lead to more sugar exposure. Synthetic fat-free or sugar-free products are not effective. Because you consume more chemicals than sugar or fat, you often eat unhealthily. Instead, stick to natural organic products to lose weight and promote health.

Loading Protein

We all made the wrong idea that too much protein would reduce the rate of eating and, thus the fat content. In fact, eating only protein food means you are depriving the body of other essential nutrients such as fats and carbohydrates. Whether you need to lose weight or not, you need a balanced diet to stay healthy and maintain optimal weight. No nutrient is good for you. You can't just focus on one type of food. You need to balance to get the power you need to lose weight.

Counting Calories

Do you think that the higher the calorie level consumed, the higher the fat achieved? If so, then you have been thinking about all the mistakes. Good nutrition doesn't always mean reducing all calories and avoiding intake. Knowing that not all calories are the same, the calorie quality that enters your body can affect your existing calories, which may surprise you. Similarly, the time of calorie intake can also affect body function. Some calories

Foods from different fruit types or foods have different effects on your body because they cause a mixed reaction in the body. You need to understand the difference between empty calories and good calories. Sticking to healthy foods is the best option when ingesting quality calories, and you don't need to control or calculate calories.

Keep Away from Snacks

Staying away from snacks does not mean completely reducing snacks. Avoid uncontrolled snacks that keep you healthy and away from unnecessary diets, but you need to control the condition of the snacks, and you'll be fine. Just like any addiction, eating less addicted food is better than a diet that completely reduces addiction today and a diet that you don't want to eat snacks tomorrow. Have a healthy nutritious meal, please stick to it, and you don't have to work hard to avoid being bitten in order to lose weight.

Low-Calorie Diet

Although in the history of weight loss programs and diets, most of them are foods with low or controlled calories. If you can't control your body to fit a particular type of diet without having to relapse or turn to junk food or other unhealthy foods, then dieting is useless. These diets often starve and reduce metabolism. Problem will

Once you start your regular diet and have a reasonable calorie in your diet, stop eating. The wise choice is to choose only foods that are commensurate with your physical needs and health requirements.

Get Rid of Dairy Products

Why do most dieters blacklist all dairy products, including ice cream, cheese, and milk? The body also needs milk, and the body needs a lot of milk. In fact, when enough calcium is supplied to the body, the body burns fat at a high rate. Lack of calcium can lead to fat production, allowing you to gain weight while losing weight. Even if it is a low-fat food, be sure to include dairy products in the shopping.

Detoxification

Detoxification is an extreme measure designed to remove toxins from the body, especially the liver. Detoxification products are designed to keep the colon clean, but according to experts, all of these products are nonsense. Your kidneys and liver are doing all the necessary cleaning work. These detox diets are juices that may contain sugar and may not be suitable for your weight level.

Skip Breakfast

Every enlightened person knows that breakfast is something you should not skip because it is crucial. You can't just eat breakfast just because you need to lose weight. Eating light food in the morning is much better than eating it completely because once you don't eat breakfast, you may eat more in the afternoon, which may eventually lead to overeating and also lead to eating food, which will increase your fat level. The more important part of the lunch and the desire to eat again before dinner are all the consequences of skipping breakfast.

Fast Food

A fast diet is more harmful to the body than a benefit. If you can't wear this dress now, you can't wear it until this weekend. Changing food intake or diet to fruit or vegetables is not good for the body system. Your diet plan should be wisely chosen.

Regardless of the modification, you will need to choose a diet plan that includes all the essential nutrients and the type of food you need, as well as a certain amount. Your goal should be to keep your body working. If you expose yourself to food without calories, your body will have a hard time burning calories once you return to a normal diet.

Go out for Meal

One day in the week, eating out a lot of calorie food is not good for your health. Restaurant foods have higher calorie content than homemade foods, and you don't even know how many calories you need to consume. Research released by the Journal of Nutrition suggests women who eat homemade food lose weight.

Not those who eat once a week at the restaurant. You can limit your meal to at least once a month, and you'll be able to strike a balance between actually losing weight and achieving the health you need.

Learn How Japanese Maintain Their Weight

The main focus of Japanese dieting is to create health rather than maintain optimal weight. However, in the process of staying healthy, one will never eat food that causes obesity or overweight. Eating habits have no restrictions on your meal. Because there is no disease, the Japanese diet focuses on maintaining health, optimal weight, and enhanced immune function. The Japanese maintain their weight through practices that can be accepted by anyone. These methods have been around for centuries, and you might consider one of the following ways to stay healthy and maintain optimal immunity.

Avoid Milk

Milk combined with any meal provides excess calcium. The disadvantage of milk consumption is that the magnesium content of the food is insufficient. There is especially a lack of milk in the Japanese diet. Even if you eat milk, you can eat it alone without eating it with any other food or food. In addition, it must be noted that dairy products slow the rate of movement of the intestines and may ultimately fail to achieve the precise level of digestion required by the body, requiring additional tissue.

Optimize Food Temperature

People around the world often ignore food temperatures, but surprisingly, the Japanese tend to focus on food temperatures. They eat warm food in cold weather and cold meals in hot weather. In the summer, cold salads, celery, and other refrigerated foods are preferred, while in the winter, meat stews and different hot soups are preferred. High energy temperatures are critical to how the body reacts to our food. It is important to consider food temperature as part of a healthy eating habit.

Healthy Snack

Unlike Western food consisting of sugar and more sugar, Japanese snacks are healthier. They have replaced most of the biscuits and chips that are consumed in the West. They prefer sunflower seeds, pumpkin seeds, dried fruits, nuts, and seaweed snacks instead of cakes and biscuits. In addition to keeping you away from too much fat, these Japanese snacks also contain micronutrients, minerals, and vitamins.

Not Every Night Is a Sweet Night

The dessert night is very good because life is very important, so you should enjoy it. However, even for your child, you must place a dessert night at least once a week. This way, you will not consume more sugar than you need. If you want something to eat, please choose any fruit instead. This one Will keep your body away from excess fat-producing substances. Avoid using ice cream, biscuits, and sweet cakes to help you lose weight and help yourself.

Rice Combination

Take a combination of rice with stronger nutrition, such as purple rice, red rice, brown rice, or even black rice. Unpolished rice is also a good source of vitamin B. The whole rice should be eaten as a supplemental meal rather than the main way to avoid the constant fluctuations in sugar in the blood. When rice is consumed too much, it will affect the glycemic index due to sugar during digestion. Due to the low starch content, the rice combination is the preferred meal in the Japanese community. Rice blends also contain fewer calories.

Seafood

Seafood offers the best combination of healthy eating, and nutrition is especially good for the body and brain. The protein in the seafood keeps you happy for a long time and does not require snacks between meals. Asians practice eating fish every day, and an important part of the diet is not to refuse. Consider using all forms of seafood every day while staying healthy while maintaining a healthy weight. Starting with ordinary fish, you can resort to other types of seafood that can expand your cooking needs while achieving good health.

Small Plates and Chopsticks

Small plates and small bowls are needed to eat small amounts of food. There are also Asians, mainly Japanese who use chopsticks. This technique is a way to avoid shoveling food to your throat. In addition, the use of chopsticks will reduce the speed of eating, and in the end, you will reduce consumption and feel good. Although the use of chopsticks and small plates may require some discipline, they are especially needed for health.

3:1 Rationing

"The vegetables you want to eat are three times more than the meat."

This is an important recommendation for replacing healthy fat with a healthy meal that contains all the essential nutrients the body needs. Fill the table with vegetables instead of meat or other fat products. Include potatoes and other green vegetables in your diet to make sure you get the right combination. Flavored vegetables will also increase your appetite. Using spices on food will help your brain prefer vegetables, and eventually, you will need more vegetables than meat. In addition, fried vegetables should be avoided as much as possible.

Soup Plan

Soup is a densely nutritious food that fills you up immediately. The incredible thing about soup is that you don't need too much. All you need is the ability to prepare healthy soup, and you are ready. Bones and vegetables are the main combinations of Japanese soup. These meals contain enough vitamins and minerals to keep your body healthy for hours. The digestion is improved due to the high temperature of the soup. Therefore, if you are having trouble digesting, especially in the winter, you can also use warm soup.

Extreme Drink

Drinks should be kept to a minimum, usually cold drinks. In fact, health professionals have emphasized the importance of avoiding cold drinks or drinking water when eating hot food or just after eating hot food. Once you avoid cold drinks, it will promote better digestion of food. Digestive enzymes are not diluted. These proteins are critical to achieving optimal levels of absorption. Enzyme activity can be increased by eating hot or green tea, which is typical in the Japanese diet. Also, consider taking the liquid 30 minutes after a meal.

Conclusion

Have you tried different ways to get your body in good shape but found that most of them are not working? Are you willing to take an exciting method that can help you to not only attain your proper weight but also experience many benefits? If you answered yes to these questions, then this ultimate guide to intermittent fasting is you. With no fluff and straight to the point the book answers all the questions that you have been asking yourself about the 16:8 intermittent fasting. Intermittent fasting is the best way to go, and this book solves all the issues and answers various questions related to intermittent fasting.

Vegan Keto Diet Meal Plan

A Step-By-Step Guide for a Keto-Vegan Diet. Meal Plan and Vegan Meal Prep That Promotes Weight Loss With a Healthy and Energetic Lifestyle

Paty Breads

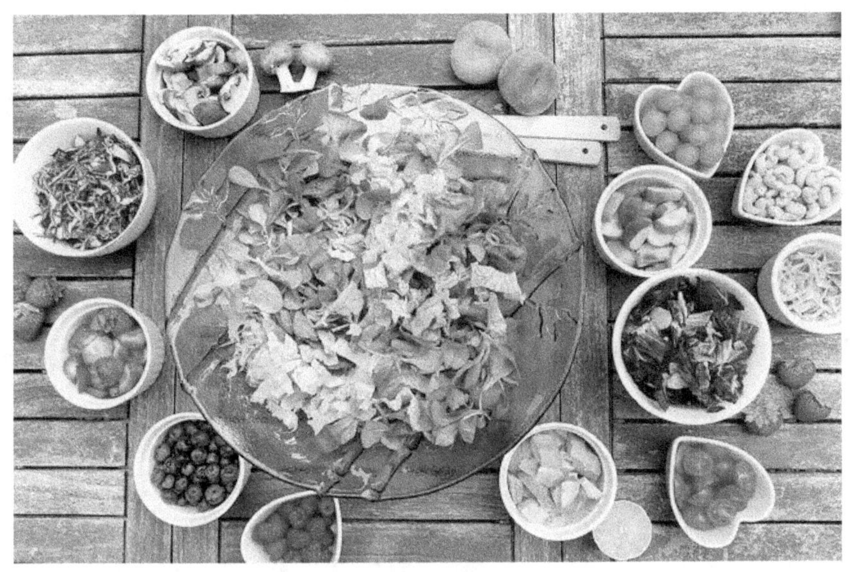

Table of Contents

The Important Things to Keep in Mind While Getting Off a Ketogenic Diet

Conclusion

truthful when it comes to the recounting of facts. As such, any use, correct or incorrect, of the provided information will render the Publisher free of responsibility as to the actions taken outside of their direct purview. Regardless, there are zero scenarios where the original author or the Publisher can be deemed liable in any fashion for any damages or hardships that may result from any of the information discussed herein. Additionally, the information in the following pages is intended only for informational purposes and should thus be thought of as universal. As befitting its nature, it is presented without assurance regarding its prolonged validity or interim quality. Trademarks that are mentioned are done without written consent and can in no way be considered an endorsement from the trademark holder.

Introduction

Congratulations on purchasing this book and thank you for doing so. This book will help you in understanding the basics of keto-vegan lifestyle and the ways in which you can incorporate it into your lifestyle with the help of Meal planning and meal prepping. This book will help you in understanding the basics of meal planning and the ways in which you can use meal prepping to your advantage.

The ketogenic diet is an effective way to fight obesity and bring wellness. It can help you in reducing and managing excess weight effectively. If you follow the ketogenic diet properly, you can also witness significant improvement in your overall health biomarkers like insulin resistance, diabetes, high blood pressure, cholesterol, and other metabolic disorders.

The world today acknowledges the impact of ketogenic diets on health and obesity. This diet has become a hot favorite of people from all walks of life around the globe. However, there are segments that have not been able to get the full benefits of this diet due to their strict dietary preferences. Vegans are also among such people.

They don't consume meat or dairy products, and hence, they feel that managing a fat-rich diet may not be possible for them. This book will help such people in understanding the concept of the ketogenic diet in detail and the ways in which even the vegans can incorporate this wonderful diet without compromising on their food preferences.

This book will explain the whole concept of the ketogenic diet in detail. From the mechanics of the diet to its specific advantages, you will get to have a look at all the aspects of this diet. However, even before that, the first section of this book will walk you through the whole battle of obesity. There are a large number of weight loss measures available in the market, and diets form a significant part of that. Having too many choices can clutter the mind, and making a definitive choice can become difficult. This book will explain the trials and tribulations a person has to go through while following a diet and the kind of end result expected. It will bring out the main reasons for failures and the ways in which the ketogenic diet addresses them.

The second section will explain the wonderful concept of the ketogenic diet and the ways in which it can help in your weight loss journey. This section would also stress on various other health benefits of following a ketogenic lifestyle.

The third section would explain the ways in which vegans can also incorporate the ketogenic diet into their lifestyle. The vegans feel that the limit food options in front of them can make it difficult to follow a ketogenic diet, which is high in fat and low in carbs. This book will give you a comprehensive list of products that can be included to get the maximum benefit of this diet.

There is no doubt that following a ketogenic diet in a vegan lifestyle can be taxing. To make it easy and convenient, this book will bring to you the ways in which meal prepping can solve the problems for you. The fourth section of the book will focus completely on meal prepping and the ways in which you can incorporate this lifestyle without having to go the extra mile. Meal prepping methods will help you in saving time and money. You'll learn that meal prepping is an easy, affordable, and time-saving way to a healthy lifestyle.

The fifth section of this book will give you a weekly meal plan spanning over four weeks so that you can plan a whole month in advance. It will also give you some easy recipes that you can try to make your meals quick and interesting.

In the end, this book will also explain the ways to manage the lost weight in the whole month so that you can really count on your success.

This book is your comprehensive guide towards incorporating vegan keto lifestyle with ease. It will give you simple tips and tricks to make this lifestyle a great success for you so that you can lose weight without having to compromise on crucial sectors.

There are plenty of books on this subject on the market, thanks again for choosing this one! Every effort was made to ensure it is full of as much useful information as possible. Please enjoy!

Chapter 1: Obesity- The Tough Problem and Even Tougher Solutions

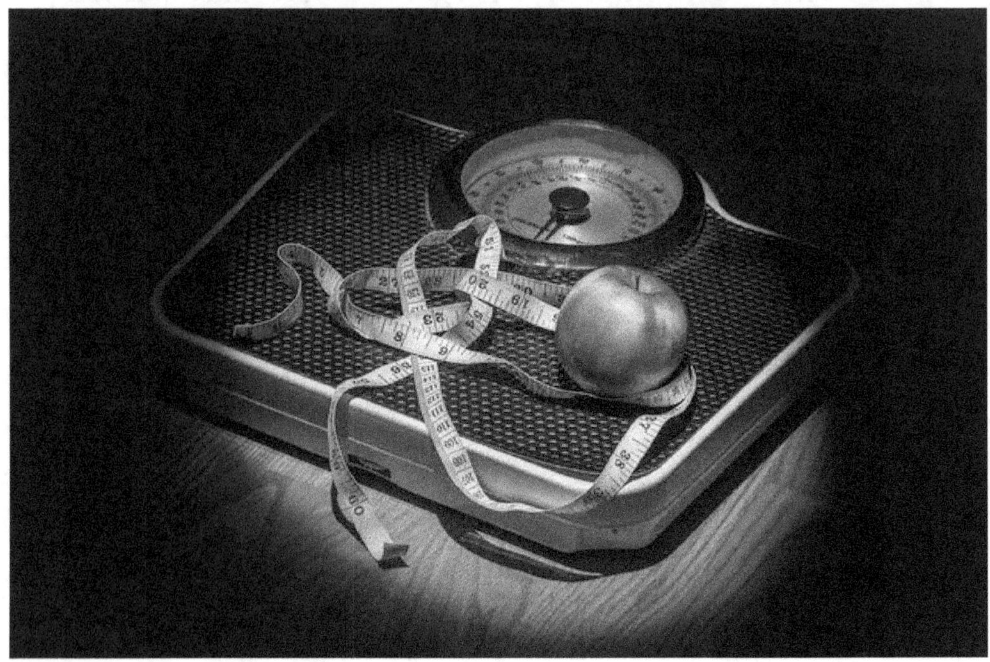

The Obesity Challenge

Obesity has emerged as the next big curse. The spread of obesity has been like a wildfire. It has taken the form of an epidemic in the past few decades. Statistics released by the World Health Organization (WHO) state that there has been a three-fold increase in worldwide obesity since 1975. The 2016 figures show that there are more than 650 million adults suffering from obesity globally. If we even start counting the people suffering from weight management issues or overweight people, then the figure can go as high as a whopping 1.9 billion.

These aren't the facts presented to scare anyone or bring any scary effect; these are real numbers that matter. What's scarier is the fact that developed countries like the US are severely affected by this problem. In fact, in the US, more than 70% of the adult population is either overweight or obese. This puts more than 2 out of every 3 people on this list. Around 39.6% of US adults are obese and are at a greater risk of getting affected by obesity-related disorders.

The big problem with obesity is that it doesn't come alone. It has its retinue. Problems like high blood pressure, diabetes, cardiovascular diseases, metabolic issues, and other such disasters strike in unison when a person gets obese. It hunts like a pack of wolves. It can pin you down and ensure that you remain pinned down to the ground forever.

This is the reason people find it extremely difficult to get out of the clutches of obesity. Most people fail to lose any significant weight at all. However, the fortunate ones who are able to lose some weight find it extremely difficult to maintain the lost weight, and that's why more than 90% of people face weight relapse.

There are 4 major ways through which people try to lose their weight:

1. **Exercise:** Exercise is a great way to maintain your current weight. However, when you are actually trying to shed several pounds of fat, this may not be the only best way to do that. To burn fat, you would need to work for several hours every day, and that would include high-intensity interval training too. It isn't practical for everyone to leave routine life aside and focus only on weight. Exercise can have a 15% impact on your weight loss, but if you are trying to get 100% from it, then maybe you're asking too much.

2. **Pills:** In this age of commerce, there are pills for almost everything. You can get several pills that may claim instant weight loss, weight maintenance, and other such things, but they don't work. There is no other sweet way of saying it. They simply don't work. You'd only end up facing the side-effects and footing the bills.

3. **Surgery:** Bariatric surgeries are advised by doctors to morbidly obese patients. However, there are certain conditions. First, the doctor must consider you a fit case for surgery. Second, they are very costly. Thirdly, the rate of weight relapse is very high even in cases of patients undertaking bariatric surgeries as managing a healthy weight is highly dependent even on your diet and lifestyle.

4. **Diet:** What we eat makes most of our weight and hence changing our eating habits, and food can bring a big

change in our weight. This is the reason the weight loss industry relies so heavily on diets. If you have the right diet, the approach towards food, and a healthy lifestyle, it is possible to lose and maintain the lost weight.

The Enigma of Weight Loss Diets

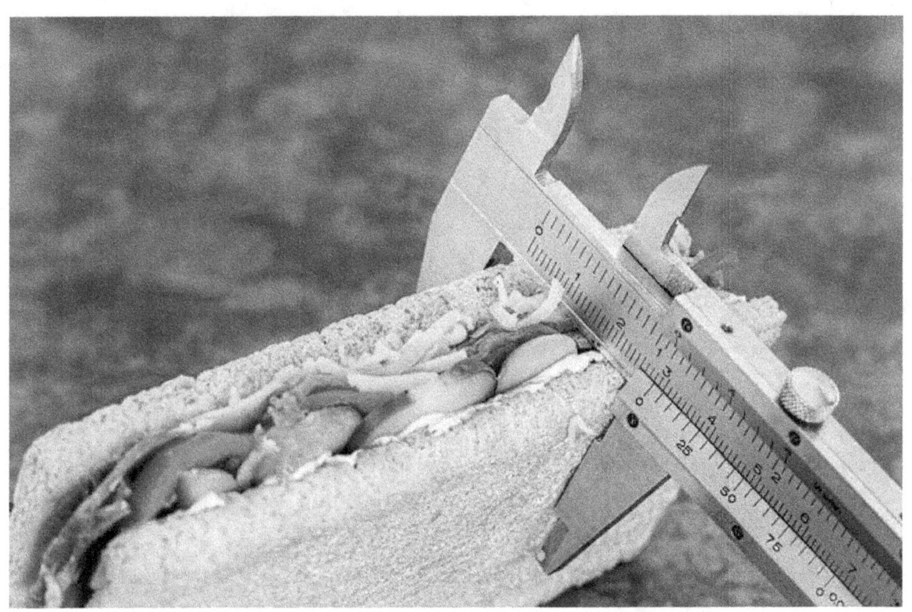

We all want to be healthy, and we all know very well that obesity is one big hurdle in the way to good health. As the rate of obesity started to rise in society, it created an urgent demand for an industry that could cater to this demand. The weight loss industry is an answer to that demand. Today, in the US alone, the weight loss industry is worth more than $72 billion.

This industry helps people in reducing and managing their weight. Of all the tricks up its sleeve, diets have been a popular medium to reduce and manage weight. A countless number of diet programs run by these companies focus specifically on weight loss.

However, it is a proven fact that, like most weight loss measures, conventional diet programs also don't work. Industry reports state that more than 80% of the people who are able to lose anywhere near 10% of their body weight regain most of it or even more in the next few months. A report published in the New York Times goes one step further and puts this percentage to be around 95.

The problem with most diet programs is that they are unsustainable and ineffective ways to lose weight.

Some major problems with diets are:
- They limit the things you can eat
- They limit the quantity of food you can eat
- They lead to insatiable hunger and cravings
- They cause mood swings and irritation

It is important to understand that food is our basic requirement. If we don't get the amount of food that our body requires, all the problems mentioned above will arise automatically. Most diet programs also put the practitioners on a calorie-restrictions. This means that not only are they restricted from eating what they want but also from eating the amount of food they want.

The First Question that comes to mind is:

Are Calorie Restrictive Diets Helpful, and Do They Lead to Weight Loss?

Initially, Yes. When a person is put on a calorie-restrictive diet, the body has to make several adjustments. It needs to lower its calorie requirements, and hence certain changes take place in the body mimicking weight loss effect. However, this weight loss is temporary, and most certainly would be back within a short span of time as actual fat burning never takes place, and the body only loses the water weight.

What is the Loss of Water Weight?

Besides providing hydration, water also plays a very crucial role in making you feel comfortable. The water in the body also helps in keeping you warm and protected against temperature fluctuations. This takes up a lot of calories. However, as you are already consuming a lot of extra calories in your daily diet, it is never a significant problem for your body.

When you go on a calorie-restrictive diet, the scenario changes drastically. Your dietician or coach would calculate your BMR and limit your calorie intake much lower than your BMR. This means that now, your body would have to survive and carry out all the functions within the restricted calorie range.

This is done to force the body to start burning fat for fulfilling the calorie deficit. However, that never really takes place as burning fat is an entirely different process that we would cover in the next chapter in detail.

When your body senses a shortage of calories, it has no other option than to manage in the limited calories available. Hence, it shuts down all the operations that are not essential for survival. This means that your metabolic rate would go down, and your body would start conserving every single calorie.

Our body tries to get rid of everything that's not very important for survival at the moment, and hence keeping the body warm or cold for comfort also comes in this list. Our body uses lots of calories in maintaining the temperature of the excess water in the body for providing extra comfort. However, as soon as there is an energy crisis, the body starts to get rid of this water. You'd lose a lot of water weight in the process, and that gives the effect of weight loss. This process takes place rapidly within a span of 1-2 weeks after beginning a calorie-restrictive diet. This is a reason people face aggressive weight loss at the beginning of their diet.

However, one remarkable thing that's common for almost everyone on a diet is that very soon they feel their weight getting plateaued. This means that very soon, they start feeling that in spite of being on a strict diet, they aren't losing any more weight. They barely manage to maintain what they have lost. They continuously need to keep upping their diets to get any weight loss effect.

Why Does This Happen?

This happens because soon, your body finds a balance. It finds a way to manage the limited number of calories you are providing it. It no longer feels the need to shed any more water weight. If you reduce your calorie intake further, you might get results, but on those calories, the body has learned the ways to manage. Although you may be stuck on a certain weight, this isn't real progress. Diets cannot go on forever, calorie-restrictive diets more so. You will have to get off the diets very soon, and as soon as you'd get off a diet, you'll see a phenomenal rise in your weight.

The Weight Relapse Conundrum

Weight relapse is one of the most common problems most people on diets face. By conservative estimates, more than 80% of people on weight loss diets experience weight relapse within a few months of getting off a diet. There are certain studies that put this estimate even close to 95%.

This happens due to several factors:

The Resurgence of Water Weight - Body's Way of Maintaining Status Quo

The body loses water weight on a diet due to a specific reason, shortage of excess calories. As soon as you get off a diet and start eating normally, that need no more exists. Your body doesn't take long to sense this change. It is always in the pursuit to provide the best conditions inside, and hence as soon as extra calories are available, water retention begins.

Another reason for the faster accumulation of water weight is the excessive presence of sugar and salt in the body. In our normal diet, we consume a lot of sugar and salt. The sugar keeps spiking our insulin levels, and that also leads to water retention. Excess sodium in the salt also causes water retention in the body. In this way, the body gets push from multiple fronts to accumulate more and more water. It also helps you feel more comfortable, and problems of excessive cold or hot flashes also go away.

All this leads to a rapid return of the water weight. People generally don't lose any real fat on most diets as fat burning is never triggered, and hence no actual weight loss is seen.

Binge Eating Takes Place- Releasing the Built-in Pressure of Temptations

If you have ever been on an actual calorie-restrictive diet or even on a diet of any specific type, you would understand the pain a dieter has to go through. It isn't the pain of not being able to eat specific things but the pain of being denied the privilege of eating those things. This pain is simply unbearable.

Human nature is rebellious. This has been programmed in our DNA to break the norms and never feel content. This is the reason behind most problems people face on a diet. You are denied the privilege of eating certain things. You may not have liked them anyway, but now that you have been denied permission to eat them, temptation starts to build for them. Their taste starts to linger in your mouth.

This isn't a problem you have to manage for a day or a week, but it can go on for weeks or months, and that is a big problem. The temptation to eat all the things denied keeps getting stronger. Your mind keeps thinking only about those things. It becomes restless.

Your mind is focused on the temptations that it is always feeling an urgent need to end the diets. It causes irritation, distraction, and lack of focus and will.

Your Body Tries to Make Up for All the Lost Food-Fighting Painful Memories

As soon as you get off the diet, your complete focus is to eat all those things all at once. Obviously, you can't do that, and hence you are on a one-point program to eat them in a short span of time.

There is always a feeling of getting released from prison, and hence, you are rewarding yourself for the punishment you have undertaken. This is one of the most dangerous feelings that leads to most problems. You have no qualms about eating all the bad things that were restricted on a diet.

Binge eating is the most dangerous thing. It will add up much more weight than you could have possibly lost through all the weight loss measures. Your mind pushes you to eat as a preventive measure. It becomes concerned about such food supply shortages coming around the way in the near future. All this puts you in a vicious trap of weight gain. There is a feeling of victimhood and a constant need for reassurance.

You are More Focused on Fulfilment than Nourishment- Caving-in to Cravings

Diets prevent you from eating many things. No doubt, most of them are bad, but habits don't change overnight. Our bodies have become habitual of eating most of those things, and when denied permission to eat, there can be strong cravings. To add to that, there is hunger, too, as you are following calorie restriction. This combination of cravings and insatiable hunger can make your condition miserable. It can make you beg for even those things that you know are certainly bad for you. Need takes over prudence in such cases. People knowing fully well that sugar and sugar-laden products are bad for them to do so. The constant hunger makes it very difficult for them to maintain the diet for long. They always feel energy-starved.

People getting off diets simply want to make up for their loss of food and taste. The idea of nourishment and gets taken over by the need for fulfillment.

This all happens due to some important reasons:

Most Diets Fail to Provide Satiety

Calorie-restrictive diets make you feel unsatisfied and hungry. When the energy intake is limited along with that, the nutrient intake also gets affected. It means you stop getting all the required macros and micros like minerals, vitamins, along with fat, protein, and carbs. This essentially means that your body is never able to feel fully satisfied. This leads to hunger and dissatisfaction. You are always prompted to break-free of the system.

A healthy ketogenic diet can help you with this. This diet helps you in getting all your macro and micronutrients.

Mental Conditioning and Preparation Isn't There

Most diets fail to take into consideration that food is our primary requirement, and it is not only a physical but psychological need too. Especially for women, when they are put on a severe calorie-restrictive routine, their hormonal cycles can become erratic. They can face serious mood swings and may also start feeling insecure. A woman's body is designed in such a way that it always needs to remain prepared for conceiving a new life. That means that it must get all the nutrients required and must never feel starved.

Several studies concerning mice have shown that their reproducing organs can shrink if they are put on a severely calorie-restricted diet.

Not only for women, but also for men, proper mental conditioning is important. If a person is put on a severely calorie-restricted diet without physical and mental conditioning, the chances of failures increase considerably.

Only willpower and determination are not enough to take your diet to success. The diet should be such that it weeds out the wrong things but puts all the required ingredients in the food. The body shouldn't feel starved. This is where the ketogenic diet wins over all other diets.

Results are So Unsatisfactory That People Feel Their Efforts Going Down the Drain

When people are going through so much in their diet, they want the results to be quick and phenomenal. However, apart from the success, you will have in the initial stages due to loss of water weight, the results would be slow, if any, at all. This creates a situation of desperation and hopelessness.

Expecting something outstanding to happen in a week or a month is not wise. There is no quick way to success. The best way out is to adopt a diet that is more sustainable and which doesn't make you feel starved all the time. Such a diet will be easy to follow, and you wouldn't find the time till results really punishing.

Apart from that, after initial weight loss, there is always a bigger challenge of maintaining that weight. With most diets, that's the most challenging part as any relaxation would mean weight relapse.

The ketogenic diet is a more sustainable way to lose weight, and it also helps you in following a healthy lifestyle forever so that weight management becomes easier. It is a proven way not only to maintain a healthy weight but also to a healthy body.

It just doesn't focus on the symptoms but the cause of the problem.

How the Ketogenic Diet Solves the Weight Loss Riddle?

One of the Biggest reasons for failures of diets is that they fail on fundamental principles. What seems to be a logical and reasonable thing doesn't work as per our expectations in our body. It has been through more than 100 million years of evolution. The ways to survive are imbibed in every cell of our body.

The first instinct of the body is to ensure survival in case there is any kind of energy shortage. If it didn't have that skill, you wouldn't be reading this now.

In the millions of years of evolution, our body has gone through several transformations. It has adapted itself to millions of things. It has learned millions more. The most important thing the body has learned is to survive, even in the toughest conditions, and wait for the bad times to pass. This led to the beginning of hibernation in many species, but the human body devised better ways to deal with it. It learned not only to survive but thrive. It developed ways to pass the bad times, and all the while keep working to avert the problems. That's why in the first few days of an energy shortage, we feel really restless, and the energy levels start going down as the days pass. But our mind is always consciously thinking about food. However, even in that condition, our body is always trying to protect its energy reserves or the fat stores as a last resort to be used when all measures fail.

That's why, whenever there is a shortage of energy supply, your body doesn't start burning the surplus fuel stored as fat immediately. It first tries to adjust all energy demands within the current supply for as long as it can. This is a measure to ensure the longest survival, and this is also the biggest hurdle in fat burning.

As a last measure, our body would burn the fat. An average person can easily survive for more than 3 months on the stored body fat itself. However, you wouldn't want to get there as of now. So, it is correct that in the complete absence of energy supply from outside, the body would start burning fat, but there are special circumstances for that, and it is difficult and painful to take that routine.

By reducing your calorie intake, you will not be able to force your body to burn fat. In fact, you will push it harder into the conservation mode, where it will do its best to reduce the need for energy. That's a reason people on a diet feel so weak, energy-starved, lethargic, and tired. It isn't the lack of energy in the body, but it's a signal to you to restore proper energy supply. The correct way to weight loss is to trigger ways of fat burning. Correct diet can definitely do that but not the one that people generally follow.

Our body can run on two different kinds of fuel:

1. Glucose Fuel
2. Fat Fuel

Both these fuels can't be used simultaneously. As long as your body is running on glucose fuel, it wouldn't burn the fat fuel, and that is the main problem in fat burning.

If you want to effectively burn fat in your body, you will have to ensure that it starts burning fat actively, and the glucose fuel supply ends completely.

If your diet is able to bring this change:

You can have actual fat burning in your body

If you bring certain changes to your diet that ensure that carbohydrate in your diet is very low and fat is high, your body would have no other option than to burn fat for energy. The energy produced by fat is cleaner and better. However, besides everything else, your body would switch to fat-burning for energy and hence whenever there is a shortage of energy, it would be able to use its own fat stores easily as it wouldn't require switching over and it wouldn't also look like an energy crunch situation requiring rationing.

This is the method that has revolutionized the weight loss segment completely. It has turned out to be an effective and easy way to reduce and manage weight.

You will never feel the energy crunch in your body

Fat fuel is cleaner, and it gives more energy per gram of content. As a comparison, 1 gram of fat produces 9 calories, whereas 1 gram of carbs only produces 4 calories. This means that even by eating smaller food portions, you will feel more energetic and stronger.

The ketogenic diets allow you to have all the macro and micronutrients in a balanced manner, and hence you don't feel energy-starved all the time. On the contrary, once you get acclimatized, you'd feel even better and more energetic.

You will not have fluctuating glucose levels

Even a lean person has fat sores that can produce more than 100 thousand calories. Whereas the total energy stored in the form of glucose is 1700-2000, this energy is stored in the form of glycogen in our muscles and liver. This means if you are on a glucose-rich diet, you will need to eat frequently, and your blood sugar levels would keep on moving up and down. When you eat, you will experience a sudden insulin spike, whereas when you haven't eaten for long like on diets, you will experience low blood sugar levels. This is a reason people on most diets feel irritated and have severe mood swings. It is our body's way of saying that it needs food to increase blood sugar levels.

There is no such problem with fat fuel. The Ketogenic diet is High in Fat and extremely Low in Carbs; this ensures that there is no fluctuation in your blood sugar levels. There are no frequent insulin spikes, and hence you feel more comfortable and at ease.

Ketogenic lifestyle can help you not only in losing weight but also in burning the fat in your body. This means that the lifestyle would help you in losing weight and staying healthy. The ketogenic lifestyle is healthy and has immense health benefits. It may look a difficult lifestyle to follow for vegans, but this book will demonstrate that it can be done easily if you put your mind and heart to it sincerely.

Chapter 2: The Miracle Called Ketogenic Diet

What Is Ketogenic Diet

Simply put, a ketogenic diet is the one that leads your body into ketosis or fat-synthesis mode.

Ketosis is the process in which your body starts to burn fat as the main fuel source. It is the most significant step towards fat loss. At this stage, you shouldn't bother about the fact that the fat comes from food or from your body, we'll get to that very soon.

On average, the diet of an American adult has 47-49% carbohydrates. This high percentage of carbohydrates is the main culprit as it prevents any kind of fat loss in your body. To understand this clearly, you must get a clear idea of the way your body metabolizes energy.

Whenever you eat food, it gets processed, and the carbs in your meal are converted into glucose. This glucose mixes in your blood and raises your blood sugar levels. Your body loves to run on glucose, as it is easy to burn fuel. Your cells can directly absorb glucose for producing energy. So, as soon as you eat something, your body senses high blood sugar levels and releases insulin to help in the absorption and storage of energy. This means every time you would consume carb-rich food, there will be an insulin spike in your blood. The insulin helps the cells in absorbing glucose. However, the cells have a limited capacity to absorb glucose, and hence the insulin then starts converting glucose to other forms to store it for future use. This is a process that needs to be carried out fast as the longer your blood sugar levels remain high, the more problems it would create.

At first, the insulin stores the excess glucose as glycogen in your muscles and the liver. However, only a limited amount of glucose can be stored in the form of glycogen. Therefore, once the glycogen stores are also full, the insulin triggers the fat cells to begin storing the remaining glucose as fat. This is the way you get the fat in your body. All the excess calories that you consume get stored as fat in this manner.

You must note one important thing here, and that's the presence of insulin. It is the main fat storage hormone in your body. As long as there is a high percentage of insulin in your body, your body would remain in fat storage mode and would never start burning the stored fat. In addition to that, as long as you keep consuming food that's high in carbohydrates, your body would never come out of fat-storage mode as there would be a constant presence of insulin in your blood, and you'd get trapped in this vicious cycle.

A ketogenic diet helps you in planning your diet in such a way that you can lose weight without having to compromise on your macros and micros. This simply means that a ketogenic diet would allow you to have a fulfilling meal that would provide you all the vital macronutrients like fat, protein, and carbs.

The ideal ratio of the macronutrients is:

Fat: 70-75%

Protein: 20-25%

Carbs: 5-10% (Whole grains, leafy greens, nuts, legumes, and fiber-rich foods)

For instance, if you consume 2000 calories a day, you'd need to have 165-170 grams of fat, 70-80 grams of protein, and less than 40 grams of carbs.

The amount of food you eat in ketogenic food goes down as fat is more compact and nutrient-dense. Even while consuming food in smaller quantities, you would be getting all the required nutrients easily.

The percentage of carbs is very low in a ketogenic diet, as its main focus is to enable your body to switch to fat fuel for energy. However, some carbs are essential because many essential vitamins, minerals, polyphenols, antioxidants, phytonutrients, etc. are obtained from them.

The percentage of protein in a ketogenic diet must always be moderate. If you are doing intense physical exercise, you can consume a little bit more protein; otherwise, you should keep the protein intake to the prescribed lower limit. The intake of protein is important as your body cannot produce it internally. The protein needs to be consumed from outside, and it is important for building muscles, and it is also used for the various repair and reconstruction purposes. However, you must always remain careful while determining the quantity of protein intake as excess protein would be utilized by the body for producing calories and would start working as carbs. This would, in fact, take you out of ketosis. Therefore, it is very important that you only consume only the required amount of protein daily.

Fat is the most important part of a ketogenic diet. Dietary fat, as well as the fat in your body, are used for producing ketones. The process of ketone metabolization is called ketosis, and ketones provide a lot of energy.

The energy produced through ketosis is clean and good.

The Science of Ketogenic Diet

Ketogenic diet began as a treatment for epilepsy. Some doctors trying to treat patients suffering from seizures found that a diet with a high percentage of fat and a very low percentage of carbs had a very positive impact on their mental growth and also stopped the seizures. The results were very promising for most of the patients, and this gave rise to more research on the subject.

The popularity of the ketogenic diet for weight loss is considerably new, keeping in view the time since when the diet has been in practice.

The weight loss science of the ketogenic diet is simple.

When your diet is very high in fat and extremely low in carbs, your body has no other option than to metabolize fats for producing energy. In the beginning, you may feel low in energy. This happens because your body is adjusting to the new fuel. First, your body would burn all the available glucose.

The glucose from food doesn't last very long as your cells have low storage capacity. When the glucose stored in the cells is over, the body starts looking for alternative energy sources.

In such a case, the glycogen stores are used. The glycogen stored in the liver can be used for this purpose. The glycogen stores can last up to 36 hours. However, after that, even the glycogen stores would get exhausted, and your body would have no other option than to begin burning the fat stores.

This leads to the release of free fatty acids that are converted by the liver into ketones. Ketones are high in energy and can be used for running your body efficiently. In fact, ketones are an excellent source of energy as they don't leave toxins as by-product contrary to glucose fuel. The process of converting the free fatty acids into ketones is known as ketosis, and that's why this diet is called a ketogenic diet.

Once your body gets into ketosis, you would start feeling full of energy. There is a lot of fat in your body, and even a small amount of fat can release a lot of energy. Fat metabolization doesn't even invoke an insulin response, and hence you stop facing the problems caused by blood sugar fluctuations.

One of the biggest problems that diets cause is unending hunger and cravings. These problems also come to a complete stop. The external and internal source of energy becomes the same for your body, and hence even if you consume food in small quantities, you wouldn't feel famished or low on energy as your body has an ample amount of fat, and it is already in the fat-burning mode.

In fact, the ketogenic diet produces the same effect on the body as fasting. When you are in a fasting state, you deny the body a chance to get glucose supply, and hence the body has no other option than to use fat for running the metabolic functions. However, fasting can be intimidating for many and may not fit into everyone's lifestyle. But there is no such problem with the ketogenic diet as it is neither punishing like fasting nor excruciatingly painful like calorie-restrictive diets as you always get the required number of calories from dietary fat and your own body's fat metabolization. In this process, there is a significant loss in body fat, and your overall health biomarkers also start improving, making you healthier.

The ketogenic diet is the best way to burn fat as it makes the fat burning process simpler for the body. It eliminates the main roadblock in front of burning fat called insulin. I've stated it earlier, too, and would like to reiterate that insulin is the biggest hurdle in burning any kind of fat in the body.

Insulin is the main fat-storage hormone. As long as you keep consuming carbs, especially refined carbs, sweets, or sweetened beverages that instantly dump too many calories into your body, the insulin levels in your body would remain significantly high. Once released, it takes at least 8-12 hours for the insulin levels to go down considerably. If you consume anything within this period, the insulin levels would get spiked again and hence would keep your body in a fat storage mode perennially.

If you want to burn fat at all, the first thing that needs to be eliminated is frequent insulin spike. The fewer carbs you consume, the lower would be the risk of the insulin spike, and hence your body would stand a better chance of fat burning.

The Impact of Ketogenic Diet on Weight Loss

The ketogenic diet did not begin as a fad diet or a weight loss diet. It began as a diet that could help in improving the neurological condition of patients suffering from epilepsy. This diet helped a lot in bringing down the occurrences of seizures in such patients. However, over the course of time, doctors realized that this diet also had several other benefits, and weight loss was only one among them.

Today, there is no doubt that the ketogenic diet can help not only in bringing down weight, but it can also help in burning fat faster than most other weight loss methods. Unlike most other diets, there is science behind these weight-loss theories, and hence you can be sure of the results if you have been following the diet correctly.

There are 4 main reasons that lead to weight loss:

Better Satiety Control

It is a proven fact that the higher the amount of cholesterol in your diet, the more cravings you will have. The reason for this is simple, the carbs are converted into glucose, and it gets processed very fast. This means that your body would need the next meal very soon. However, that doesn't happen with the ketogenic diet. It is high in protein as compared to carbs. Scientific studies have conclusively proven that the consumption of a greater amount of protein as compared to carbs leads to greater satiety. Fats and protein take much longer to get processed and keep your digestive tract engaged. This also means that the release of the hunger hormone Ghrelin decreases in your gut, and hence, you have a lower appetite.

When you are relying heavily on a refined carb-rich diet, snacking frequently in between your meals becomes a compulsion as there would be frequent food cravings. As soon as you consume a carb-rich diet, your blood glucose increases, and your insulin levels go up. However, it doesn't last long, and your blood glucose levels go down very soon. This leads to excessive cravings.

A fat and protein-rich diet, on the other hand, faces no such issue, and hence you can easily pass on from one meal to another without feeling the need to have snacks.

Lower appetite also means that your food consumption also goes down, and that also contributes to weight loss.

Fat building stops and fat breaking begins-Lipolysis

The most significant thing that a ketogenic diet does to your body is that it begins the 'Lipolysis' process. Lipolysis is the event in which your body stops storing fat anymore and starts breaking down the fats and other lipids in the body to release free fatty acids.

In simple terms, this means that your body comes out of the fat storage mode. The biggest problem with most weight loss methods is that although they are trying to help you in losing weight, they are never really able to stop the body from storing fat. However, the ketogenic diet is able to do just that in a very simple way.

Your body actively targets the fat stores, and your cholesterol and triglyceride levels start to go down significantly. If you have been worried about your high cholesterol and triglyceride levels and lipid management, this is the diet for you.

The more actively your body starts to target your fat stores, the faster will be your progression towards fat loss.

However, here, you must understand one important point. Fat loss may not always lead to weight loss as both are an entirely different thing. Another important thing to note is that increasing weight is not a bad thing as long as your waist size is going down.

When your body is in the process of ketosis, it starts burning the fat stores in your body. The adipose tissues or the fat deposits at your waist, thighs, and hips get targeted the most as the fat deposits are high at these places. However, although the fat is voluminous in size, it doesn't have much weight.

This means that although your fat may be burning, you may not notice significant improvement on the weighing scale. If you are also witnessing this, you may be ignoring another important factor, and that is muscle buildup.

The ketogenic diets are not only high in fats, but they are also high in protein. This means that if you do regular exercise, you will bulk muscles, and that's why it is a favorite diet of people in the bodybuilding community.

Therefore, all the while, the muscle mass in your body may be going up, which may have caused your weight to go up. This also means that you will get muscular and stronger.

So, if you are trying to gauge your progress, you must do that on both scales. Measure the circumference of your waist and hips and also weigh yourself to get a clear picture.

Increased Calorie Expenditure

There are specific reasons that our body loves carbs. It is very easy to burn and use as glucose. The same cannot be said about fat and protein. The transition is tough for the body. In the beginning, your body first tries to use every measure to stick to glucose. Once the glucose stores are depleted, the body begins metabolizing the remaining protein. The amino acids in the body are converted, and the body even tries to break down muscles for producing energy. However, excessive catabolization is counter-productive, and hence the body has to use fat as energy.

Conversion of fat into ketones takes up a lot of energy, and hence, the calorie expenditure in your body increases even if you are maintaining a sedentary lifestyle.

This means that your body would have to burn more calories, even for performing similar actions. This leads to faster weight loss.

Metabolic functions improve

The ketogenic diet has a very profound impact on your metabolic functions. The absence of glucose in the body gives your metabolic functions a great jolt. Burning glucose is simple, and hence most metabolic functions remain in a relaxed state. However, the ketogenic diet forces the body to start burning fat and protein for energy. The metabolic functions that had become slow due to issues like insulin resistance, high blood sugar, or blood sugar fluctuations also improve.

Most of the metabolic functions start to react actively, as more calories are being used to produce the same amount of energy. This also accelerates your metabolic functions, and you start to lose weight faster.

The health benefits of the ketogenic diet are far and wide. It is a diet that can help in the overall improvement of health. Most of us are plagued by the misconception that our poor health is a result of obesity. On the contrary, it is the other way around. Poor health is the cause of increasing fat stores in the body. When the blood sugar control in your body becomes weak, when your body has poor fat regulation and when metabolic disorders are attacking you left, right, and center, obesity is bound to affect you big time. Obesity is a symptom that the problems are getting out of hand and not the main cause of the problem in the first place.

A proper ketogenic diet can help you in preventing these risk factors, and hence weight management would become much simpler than you can think.

Some of the Important Health Benefits of Following a Ketogenic Diet are:

Improved Insulin Sensitivity and Blood Sugar Management

The biggest factor that affects our overall health and also our weight is uncontrolled blood sugar. This is a problem that also gives way to diabetes and other pancreatic disorders later on. One of the most important things that lead to poor sugar control is excessive reliance on refined carbs and sugar. Modern-day diet has become such that the use of refined carbs and refined sugar has increased a lot in it. These things bring a sudden rise in our blood sugar and insulin levels and then also deplete very fast. Excessive consumption of refined carbs also gives way to food cravings. You rely heavily on snacking and frequent meals to get your blood sugar-fix. However, deep down, that's a very dangerous thing, and it slowly starts making your body insulin resistant.

It means that the more frequent meals you have, the lower you will be able to fulfill your body's current energy demands. Your cells would start getting overexposed to insulin and hence would stop reacting actively to insulin signals. This would mean that although you would be eating food, your body wouldn't be able to absorb the glucose derived from that food. At this stage, this disease is known as diabetes.

A ketogenic body deprives your body of carbs to a great extent. This means that the exposure of cells to insulin becomes really low. You rely heavily upon fat, and that produces an alternative source of energy known as ketone that is further broken down to ATP that helps in running the body. Your body would be able to run efficiently without having to generate an insulin response. This helps in improving the insulin sensitivity in your body, and the blood sugar management in your body gets better. If a person suffering from diabetes is put on a strictly controlled ketogenic diet under the supervision of a doctor, great results can be achieved in terms of sugar control.

Blood sugar management can be the solution to most health problems as it is also spreading like a big epidemic. Currently, there are more than 110 million adults in the US alone suffering from prediabetes and diabetes. Especially the people suffering from prediabetes can get benefited more as the problem is still under progression, and it can be fully reversed.

Diabetes is among the top 5 causes of preventable deaths in the US. If proper blood sugar management can be achieved, a lot of lives can be saved.

Better Lipid Control

Poor lipid control is also a major cause of concern these days. People suffer from all sorts of cholesterol issues, and that affects their hearts adversely. It is more than common to find people with heart problems with inflated levels of bad cholesterol (LDL), VLDL, total cholesterol, and triglycerides. High levels in these areas can poorly affect the functioning of your heart.

We usually put the blame on higher lipid levels on fats. However, we seldom realize the main culprit even here is sugar. The carb-rich diet and poor eating habits lead to insulin resistance in the body. It can lead to clogging up of arteries and would prevent fat burning too.

A ketogenic diet can help you in getting over these issues as it helps in reducing your bad cholesterol (LDL), VLDL, total cholesterol, and triglycerides. Not only this, your good cholesterol levels start increasing significantly.

When you follow a ketogenic diet, your body stops running on a glucose fuel and begins lipid synthesis. This means the triglycerides are the first to get attacked as they are used as a fuel. You'd find that after a few weeks of a ketogenic diet, your lipid levels would improve considerably. Your heart would become much safer and healthier.

Improved Cognitive Abilities

This is also an interesting aspect of following a ketogenic diet. This diet was designed originally for improving cognitive abilities in patients suffering from epilepsy. There have been extensive studies demonstrating the fact that this diet can provide better relief in such cases. The brain basically runs on glucose fuel. However, it can run better on ketones as it causes much lover oxidative stress and chronic inflammation. Following a healthy ketogenic diet can give your brain a great boost.

Improved Longevity

Our longevity is a sum total of our overall health biomarkers. If your insulin sensitivity is great, your body is processing the lipids fine, your heart is working smoothly, your brain is functioning fine, and your liver is not under pressure, you will automatically have a better chance of longer life. This is what comes naturally to you when you follow a ketogenic diet.

This diet helps in improving your overall health. It addresses the fundamental health issues in the body so that it can work more efficiently.

Although the ketogenic diet has great health benefits, people feel intimidated by this diet. Their apprehensions are about the limited number of food choices available to them on this plan. The dependence on fat increasing and the carb intake becomes very low.

People are worried that this lifestyle would be very difficult for them to follow.

If this diet plan was already not very difficult to follow, it becomes more so when you have to follow it in a vegan lifestyle as your food choices get severely restricted.

People feel that it is difficult to follow.

It is very costly.

It would consume a lot of their time.

The next chapter would explain the ways in which a ketogenic lifestyle can be followed easily while being a vegan. You wouldn't have to compromise on your vegan principles to get all the amazing health benefits of the ketogenic diet.

The next chapter would explain in detail the things you can eat and the ways in which this lifestyle can be used for reaping all the health benefits.

In fact, while being a vegan, it gets even easier for you to transition to a ketogenic lifestyle and get off it without facing side effects. When people following regular diets adopt a ketogenic lifestyle, they encounter a lot of problems, including sugar withdrawal symptoms. When they get back to their regular eating style, then also the transition becomes difficult for them as their bodies develop high insulin sensitivity.

For vegans, it is a much simpler transition as there are a lot of leafy greens in their lifestyle already, and they prevent any kind of problem.

Chapter 3: Veganism- A Great Way to a Healthy Life

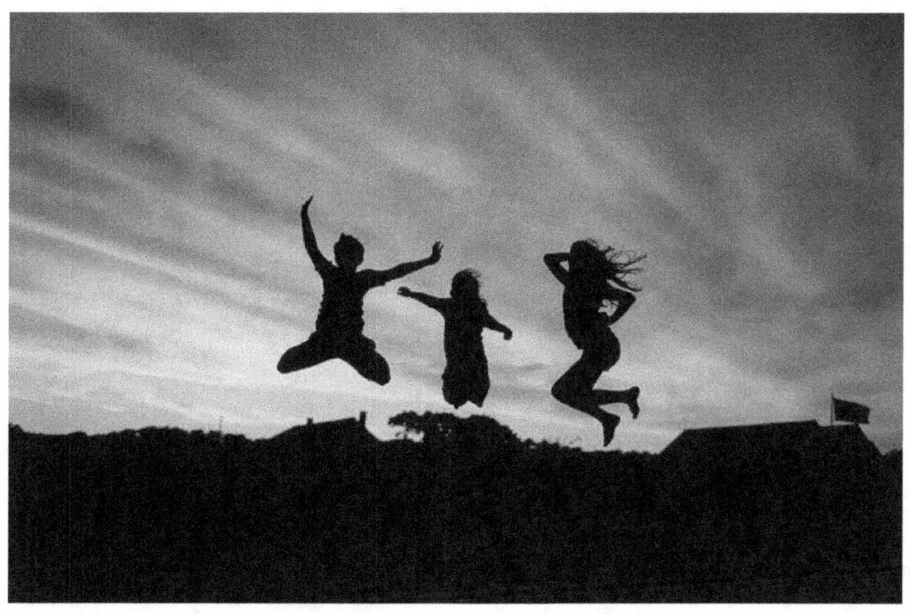

What Is Veganism?

The idea of veganism is simple; your diet would only comprise of food items derived from plants. Although veganism is becoming a popular choice these days due to rising health concerns, it isn't a very easy lifestyle to follow.

Being vegan doesn't only mean leaving non-vegetarian food like vegetarians but completely shunning any type of food product obtained from animals, even dairy products. This may look like a very restrictive dietary choice, but it is being widely followed by people and has great health benefits.

The idea of veganism was propagated by the people who chose to take a moral stand for cruelty against animals. Animals are slaughtered in millions, and even the ones that are reared for milk and eggs don't live in very hospitable conditions. All these things prompted people to lead a life that was free from all kinds of animal products.

However, this lifestyle gained even greater traction when people saw the immense health benefits of the vegan lifestyle. A complete plant-based lifestyle not only provides an ample amount of fiber to you but also gives you the required macro and micronutrients. Some people raise their concern over high starch content in the plant-based diet and the number of carbs you can consume. However, going vegan also means that you will be eating a whole lot of fiber too. This fiber nullifies the effect of starch to a great extent and keeps your digestive tract clean.

This lifestyle can help you lose weight faster than some of the popular weight-loss diets like Atkins or Paleo diets. The best thing about this lifestyle is that you can easily and effortlessly keep losing weight without having to feel starved.

The calorie content in vegetables is so low that even if you eat to your heart's content, you will remain below your daily quota. Not only this, the fibers that you consume in the process would keep you feeling fuller for much longer than any other carb-based diet.

The shift towards veganism has also been due to the dangerous impact of eating animal-based products. Despite the regulations, meat-based products can never have the assurance of being fresh, disease-free, and antibiotics free. Even dairy products come laden with similar problems. Veganism seems to be a simple yet effective alternative to the problem.

Studies have also confirmed that plant-based diets are especially very effective in several chronic illnesses. You can follow this lifestyle if you are really concerned about lowering the risk of some of the major health risks.

Veganism can be very helpful in:

Effectively Managing Type 2 Diabetes: There are several studies that vouch for the fact that you can manage the risk of type 2 diabetes much better if you are following a plant-based diet. Plants based food is low on the glycemic index and hence invokes negligible insulin response. The high fiber content in this diet helps in suppressing the frequent ghrelin release. You are able to manage your hunger and weight better with this diet.

Reducing the Risk of Cardiovascular Diseases: Heart diseases are at the top when it comes to health issues that cause the highest number of preventable deaths in the US. A plant-based diet can be very helpful if you want to fight heart diseases effectively. A high number of antioxidants, polyphenols, and other nutrients help in reducing chronic inflammation and oxidative stress. This goes a long way in ensuring heart health. The high amount of fiber is the diet is also very helpful, and this diet also helps in bringing down insulin resistance. All these things cumulatively help in lowering the risk of heart diseases.

Lowering the Risk of Cancer:

Cancer is becoming a greater concern these days as it is taking more and more people under its clutches. Studies have proven that a plant-based diet can be a helpful step towards preventing the onset of cancer in the body.

Veganism is a healthy lifestyle choice. There is no doubt that for some people, transition into veganism can be easy. People coming from Asian countries may find it relatively easy to adapt to this lifestyle as many people from that region are essential vegetarians. It is a part of their religion and culture. However, people following a completely western lifestyle may find it a bit harsh in the beginning. However, there is greater hope now as more vegan options are available these days as compared to the past. You can even by food products even at stores that would have fully vegan markings.

It is a small amount of sacrifice in the beginning to adopt a vegan lifestyle, but it is a healthy choice for a lifetime as it can help you in minimizing the risk of diseases several times. It is ethically, morally, and environmentally a great step.

We have already discussed the overall positive impact veganism can have on health. Given below are some of the specific health advantages that you can get by adopting this lifestyle.

Increases Satiety and Suppresses Hunger

The plant-based food is rich in dietary fiber. It is also voluminous, and while it carries comparatively very few calories. Hence, you can eat it in large quantities without having to worry about calorie management. This means you will be consuming a lot of it every day. Most part of the fiber in the plant-based diets is indigestible that sits for long and helps you in feeling fuller even several hours after your meal. This means that you wouldn't start feeling hungry or wouldn't have food cravings frequently. This is really very helpful when you are trying to lose weight. Cravings and hunger are some of the biggest hurdles in limiting calorie intake or following a healthy lifestyle. This gets taken care of automatically when you follow a vegan lifestyle.

Excellent Nutrition

The plant-based diet is rich in antioxidants, polyphenols, phytonutrients, minerals, and vitamins. These are some of the things that are difficult to find in animal-based diets. Following a vegan lifestyle, you can be sure that you would be getting all the required nutrients in ample quantities.

Helps Controlling Calorie Intake

Calorie intake goes low automatically when you follow a plant-based diet as it is voluminous but low on calories. Even if you stuff a lot of plant-based food, you'd still be lower in calorie consumption as compared to an animal-based diet.

High Fiber Improves Digestion

Fiber-rich food is excellent for your digestion system. One of the best things about high fiber food is that it doesn't get processed quickly, like high-carb diets. Soluble fiber forms a gel-like solution and helps in proper absorption of nutrition. The indigestible fiber helps in cleaning your digestive tract and intestines thoroughly as it comes out unprocessed. Both these fibers help in keeping your digestive system robust. If your digestive system is strong, you will have a stronger immune system, and it would become easier for your body to manage weight.

Increases Longevity

The plant-based diet is rich in minerals, vitamins, antioxidants, phytonutrients, etc. They help in fighting chronic illnesses and ensure that your metabolic function remains robust. All these factors help a lot in increasing your longevity. Not only this, lower inflammations and a high intake of antioxidants also ensures that you have better anti-aging effects.

Better Hormonal Balance

One of the biggest problems with animal-based diets is that they can cause greater damage to your hormonal balance. It is an open secret that the animals get injected hormones and anti-biotics for faster and robust growth. Through them, they ultimately end up in our system.

For instance, consumption of too much animal fat can raise the estrogen levels in our body alarmingly. It is a proven fact that excessive estrogen levels can be a factor for the growth and development of cancer in the body.

The anti-biotics that ends-up in our system through animals is another problem.

A plant-based diet can provide a complete respite from this problem.

Relief in Arthritic Pain

Studies have proven that chronic inflammation is responsible, to a great extent, behind arthritis pain. Hence, if you consume a plant-based diet, you will be able to consume a lot of antioxidants that can help in relieving arthritic pain.

Lowers Blood Sugar Levels

A plant-based diet is exceptionally good for lowering blood sugar levels as it invites very low insulin response and doesn't spike your blood sugar levels. The fiber in the diet also keeps your gut engaged for longer, and hence, the ghrelin release or the release of the hunger hormone also remains limited. All these things help in safely managing your blood sugar levels. If you are a diabetic, this diet can be a boon for you.

Improvement in Kidney Function

The kidney function is also greatly connected to your blood sugar levels. If blood sugar management is better in your body, your kidneys will be able to function in a much better way.

Enhances Mood and Helps in Controlling Mood Swings

The plant-based diet is known for inducing positivity and joy in life. It keeps you feeling refreshed and doesn't make you lethargic, unlike animal-based diets. Better blood sugar and hunger control also ensure that you don't have abrupt mood swings caused by excessive food cravings.

Now we know that both the Vegan diet as well as ketogenic diet are great for our health and lead to weight loss. If we can club both the diets, we can have a better way to manage our health. However, people have concerns that veganism and ketogenic diets are two completely different diet programs. A vegan diet would primarily be a carb-rich diet, as most plant-based products have high starch content. Whereas the ketogenic diet advises very low carb content and high-fat content. There is no doubt in the fact that finding fat in a plant-based diet can be challenging and that too, at such a high rate.

You may feel this to be a sticky situation, but if you look at it differently, you will find that it is a winning combination.

The ketogenic diet requires you to restrict sugar completely and eat a lot of fat. However, this kind of liberty mostly gets misused. People start consuming all kinds of fats without considering the quality of the fat. Dependence only on fat also makes the diet monotonous, and people at times find it difficult to follow as it doesn't suit the taste buds. There is a doubt that the eating options get limited when you get on a specific type of diet. Almost similar problems plague people who are trying to follow a vegan diet. They think that simply because they are consuming a plant-based diet, they don't need to watch anything. This eventually causes more problems than they can think of. If you start consuming carb0-rich vegetables, even in a plant-based diet, you can't expect your weight to go down. Your choice of food needs to be prudent and judicious.

When you are trying to follow a keto-vegan diet, the biggest challenge in front of you would be to manage the macros carefully. There are ways to get fat, but when it comes to protein, things get a bit tricky. There are many legumes that can provide ample protein, but they are also rich in carbs. This means if you are even trying to partially fulfill your protein quota, you will exceed your carbs limit for the day. The solution is to find a vegan source of protein that fulfills your needs without increasing the carb intake. However, the solution to this problem lies in protein-rich products like tofu, tempeh, and soy yogurt.

Following a proper keto-vegan diet can help you in getting the best of both the worlds.

Can Vegans Follow Ketogenic Diet?

There are plenty of options available even in plant-based diets that can help you in consuming fat-rich food. If you are consciously following a keto vegan diet, you will be more aware of the kind of vegetables you consume. Your focus would be more towards non-starchy leafy green and not on carb-rich potatoes.

This is correct that both diets have their definite principles, but they can be made to work together. If you follow a keto-vegan diet properly, you can be sure of experiencing faster weight loss, and you would also be able to overcome most health challenges. The best thing about following a keto-vegan diet program is that once you get off a keto diet, you will be able to maintain your weight very easily. On a keto diet, your body becomes very sensitive to glucose, and your insulin sensitivity improves considerably. If you get back to a normal diet after keto, you will gain much faster than before as your body would be processing sugar much better.

The best way to get off a keto diet is to follow something like a Mediterranean diet where your vegetable intake is higher, and sugar intake is minimal. This is natural in a plant-based diet, and hence the transition would be very easy for you.

Therefore, clubbing both the diets together would mean that you will be taking out the bad things from both the diets and would be keeping on the good things consciously. This would give you faster and better results.

As far as vegan food items that support keto are concerned, the list is pretty long, and hence you can be sure that you would get a lot of variety.

From getting proteins to your fat, the plant-based diet can give you plenty of options to choose from.

Going vegan is a choice. However, it can be a tough choice if you have been following a traditional diet in the past. As much as the challenges are regarding the diet, there are certain social and personal challenges too.

Going vegan means that you might face problems in dining out. Your food choices may get limited while you are traveling, and you may find problems in finding the proper food of your liking. You may also face problems in attending parties and social events as you may feel left out of missing on the fun with others. Things can also get awkward while trying to explain your food choices to your friends and family. However, these are minor challenges that you may have to face sometime.

While Dining Out

It is always best to find places to dine out, which offer vegan food. If you are dining out with friends, it might look tempting to go with the flow once in a while, but this temptation must be curbed as it can take the form of a habit very soon. Even if the place doesn't serve vegan food, salads are always safe and can be consumed anywhere.

While Traveling

Traveling is a part of our life. We have to go out for work or due to social obligations. When traveling, it isn't always possible to carry food, especially if you are going on a long trip. Preparation is the best way out in such cases. Always research well about the place you are going to visit. Try to find the places where you can get vegan food or plan in advance the things you can readily get to eat. This will help you in saving a lot of time and fuss in a new place.

Being Frank with Your Food Choice

If you want to save a lot of trouble, it is always in your best interest to disclose your food choices to your close friends and family. The more you try to remain private about it, the more inconveniences you'll have to face, and there will be several awkward moments in the process. Tell them about your food choices and your rationale behind it. This will help them in understanding your perspective and also in preparing in advance when inviting you for food.

Some Very Important Things to Keep in Mind While Following a Keto-Vegan Diet

Although the keto-vegan diet is great, and it combines the best of both the worlds, there are certain things that you need to be careful about while following this diet plan.

Watch Out for Some Vitamin and Mineral Deficiencies

One of the biggest problems that keto-vegans face is that they miss out on many essential vitamins and minerals that come from animal products. For instance, Vitamin B-12 is an essential vitamin that comes from animal products like meats, dairy products, cheese, eggs, etc. but, vegans don't have any of it. This can lead to vitamin B-12 deficiency, which can be very damaging. Its deficiency can cause amnesia, dizziness, and even memory loss. Deficiencies of other vitamins such as Vitamin D and K2 are also common.

The same goes for minerals, as well. Vegans can be deficient in zinc, iron, and calcium.

Although the plant-based foods are rich in rich in antioxidants, getting enough omega 3 fatty acids always remains a challenge for vegans. Although they can get it from nuts, people generally don't eat those many nuts in their daily life to fulfill their daily requirements.

Focus on Fortified Foods, Whole Foods, and Enhance Nutrient Availability

As discussed above, vegans can miss out on many vitamins and minerals that may cause problems in a healthy life. The best way to solve this problem is to consume fortified foods that have been enriched with certain vitamins and minerals. In this way, you will be able to overcome a big hurdle in your way.

Whole foods are also good for maintaining a healthy vegan life. It has been noticed that vegan people simply look for vegan options and don't care much about the aspect of the overprocessing of food. There are so many products are available in the market, specifically targeting the vegans that are so overprocessed that they will kick you out of ketosis the instant you eat them. If due attention is not paid, you wouldn't be able to achieve ketosis, and hence your weight loss goals would remain unachieved.

It is always the best to focus as much as possible on whole foods as they have a lot of fiber, they are low on carbs, and they also contain important minerals. The more a food item gets processed, the higher would be its carb content, and lower would be its fiber content. This should be avoided.

Another important thing to note is that you can easily increase the nutrient value of food products by fermenting and sprouting them. This should be followed as much as possible. This will enable you to have more value from your food items.

Don't Underestimate the Importance of Supplements

The vegan keto lifestyle is very healthy, but you may still lack in certain areas. Your body may miss protein, certain vitamins, and minerals, as well. To counter this problem, it is important that you take the help of certain supplements. You can go for vegan options as there is no need to compromise on your principles, but completely ignoring the need for supplements wouldn't be prudent.

Managing the Keto Flu

Keto flu is common and does affect the body in the beginning. There is nothing to worry but proper management of flu-like symptoms arising is important.

Flu-like symptoms that arise at the beginning of a keto diet are known as keto flu.

While you are consuming a regular carb-rich diet, your body runs on glucose. Ketogenic diet pushes your body hard to switch the fuel supply from glucose to fat, and that causes some adverse reactions.

This happens because when you are consuming too much sugar, the water retention in your body is high. When you begin a low-carb diet, the body, especially the kidneys, start dumping water and electrolytes along with it. This causes dehydration.

There may be:

- Nausea
- Fatigue
- Constipation
- Irritability
- Headache
- Muscle cramps
- Dizziness
- Difficulty in sleeping

If you face these challenges, there is nothing to worry about as these symptoms would subside soon.

To deal with them:

Stay hydrated

Your body will be dumping water, and a simple solution to that problem is to remain hydrated. Drink a lot of water.

Take electrolytes

Your body will be losing on minerals while it dumps water, and hence it is always better to take electrolytes to fulfill the mineral deficiency. The major minerals you lose are magnesium, potassium, and sodium. You can easily replenish them with electrolytes.

Take rest

It is important to rest properly as it would give your body the required time and energy to recover.

Eat fiber-rich food

Consuming fiber-rich food on a keto-vegan diet wouldn't be a problem as the majority of food is full of fiber. The fiber content will help you in fighting with constipation and diarrhea

The Macros

It is important that you first understand the equation of macros clearly so that following a keto-vegan path becomes easier.

Carbohydrates

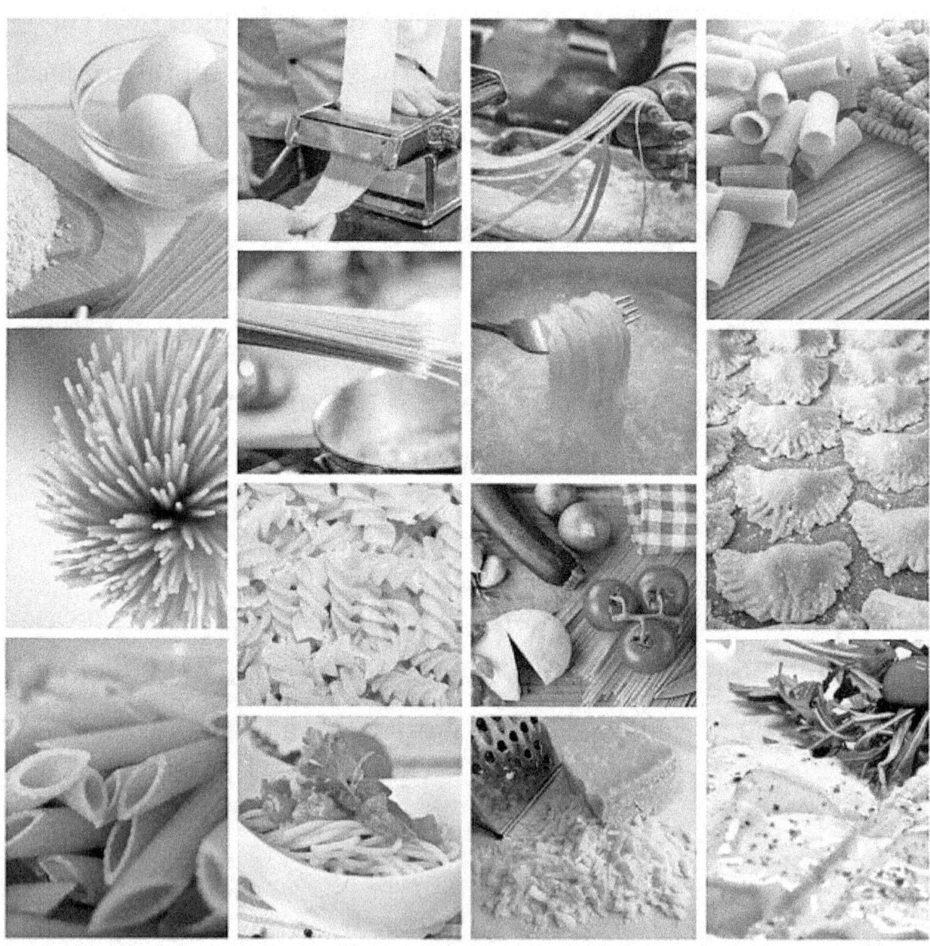

This is one of the most controversial macronutrients in a ketogenic diet but also an essential one in a vegan diet, and hence, discussing it is important. You will need to limit your carb intake below 50 grams per day, and it can be a challenging task while being vegan.

Most of the food items in the vegan list have some amount of carbs, and hence, finding a middle ground is important.

The best way out is to choose non-starchy leafy green vegetables as their carb content is very low, and they are nutrient-dense.

You should completely avoid high starch vegetables like potato and sweet potato as they can kick you out of ketosis due to their high sugar content.

As far as fruits are concerned, consider high-fat fruits like avocadoes, olives, and berries. They are low on the glycemic index and provide nutrients.

For getting protein and fat, you can turn to healthy nuts like the Macedonian nuts and almonds. However, you must avoid nuts that have very high carb content like cashew nuts.

The correct calculation of carb content in food products is very important. You need to keep your daily carb content under 40 grams. You can keep the green leafy vegetables out of this calculation because the carb content in them is very low. You can easily consume as many leafy greens as you want without fear.

While consuming carbs from other sources, you must read the product labels carefully. You have to keep in mind that your net carbohydrate intake remains under 40 grams. The easiest way to do this is to read the label and find out the total carb content and the fiber content. Deducting the fiber content from total carb content will give you a clear calculation of net carb content. For instance, you have taken nuts that have a total carb content of 40 grams. The fiber content in those nuts is 30 grams. Then the net carb content would be 10 grams. In this way, you will be able to assess the actual carb content in a day.

The better you manage your carb intake, the easier it would become for your body to maintain ketosis.

Some good carb sources are:

Low Carb Vegetables

- Cucumber
- Collard greens
- Asparagus
- Swiss Chard
- Mushroom
- Spinach
- Bell Pepper
- Kale
- Green Beans
- Cauliflower
- Cabbage
- Squash
- Eggplant

- Broccoli
- Onions
- Tomatoes
- Garlic

Although I have mentioned several times that refined carbs should be avoided completely. You must strictly avoid the following at all costs:

- Sugar
- Refined Flour
- Fruit juice
- Pasta
- Bread
- Tortillas
- Chips
- White rice
- Carrots
- Corns
- Potatoes and sweet potatoes
- Cereals
- Starchy vegetables
- All food items that have refined flour and added sugar

Fats

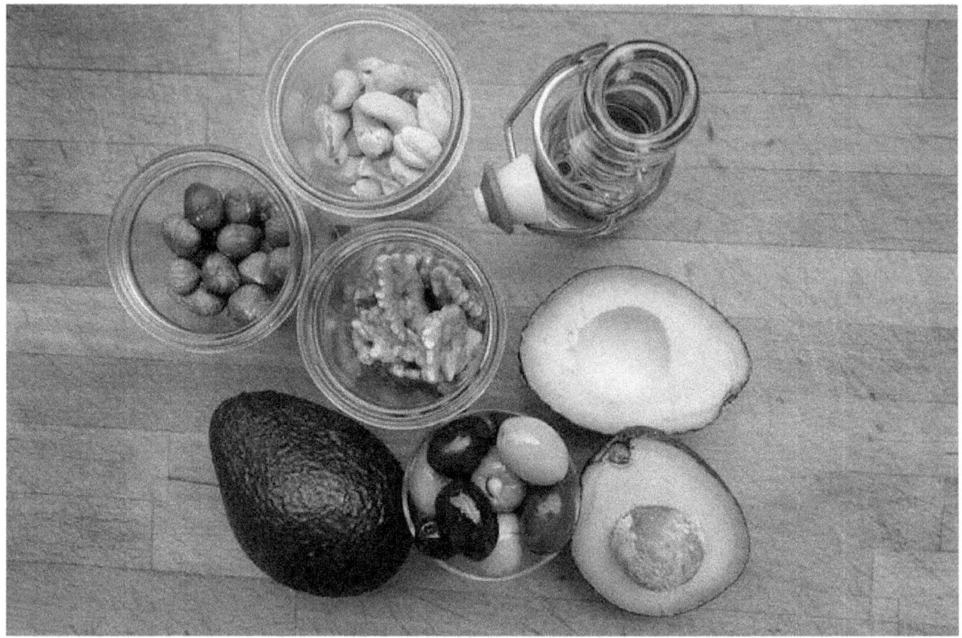

All things are not created equal, and this is true even for fats. While you need to consume fat in large quantities, this doesn't mean you can have any kind of fat. It is correct that your options for fat intake are limited, yet you must decrease your reliance on vegetable fats. Most part of your fat must come from healthy sources like olive oil, macadamia nut oil, coconut oil, almonds, avocadoes, sesame seeds, etc. These fats have high nutritional value, and they help your body to remain in ketosis. The most important thing is to ensure that the fats you consume are minimally processed. The more processing they get, the higher will be the degradation in their nutrient value.

Some good fat sources are:

Oils

Olive Oil: This oil is rich in oleic fatty acids and has a high quantity of Omega-3 fatty acids. It has amazing antioxidant properties and helps in fighting chronic inflammations too. It is a very healthy fat to be included in your keto diet.

Avocado Oil: This oil is also high in oleic acid and has high percentages of omega 9 fatty acids. You can also get vitamins A and E along with carotenoids and magnesium through this oil.

Coconut Oil: Coconut oil is rich in many things and produces an antibacterial, antifungal, and antiviral effect. It can even be used for treating yeast infections. It improves your heart health and can bring fast weight loss effects.

MCT Oil: This oil is known as a super fuel. It means medium-chain triglyceride (MCT), and it is sourced from coconut oil. Your body can use this oil as a direct fuel source, and it speeds up the process of ketosis. It improves weight loss, reduces your cholesterol levels, improves calorie combustion rate, improves gut health, and improves blood sugar levels.

Sesame Seed Oil: It is an easily available oil that's high in Vitamin B, D, and E. It is also rich in minerals like calcium, copper, phosphorus, and zinc. It boosts metabolism and prevents the development of several problems.

Nuts

Walnuts: These are high in monosaturated and polyunsaturated fats along with omega 3 fatty acids.

Almonds: These nuts are a great source of fat, protein, and fiber. These are rich in vitamins, minerals, and healthy fats.

Macadamia Nuts: These nuts can help in lowering cholesterol and triglyceride levels in your body. They also help in preventing cell damage.

Proteins

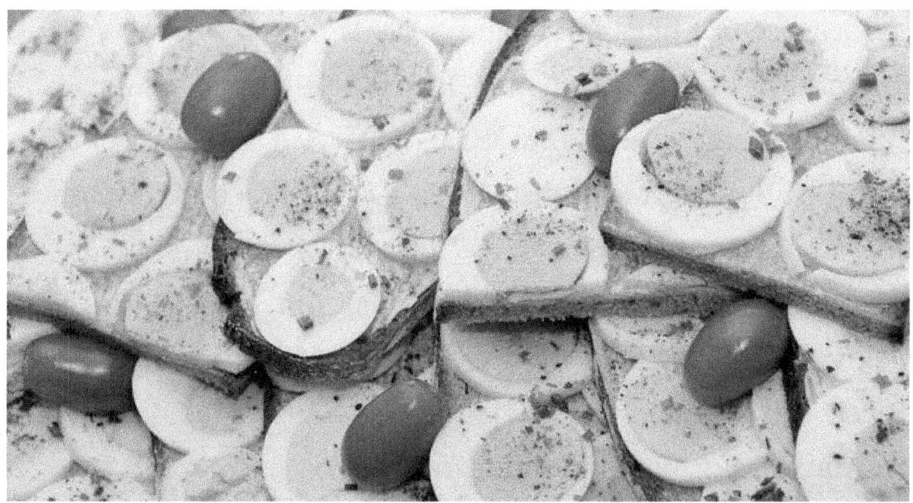

Although ketogenic diets focus more on fats, the role of proteins can never be ignored. You should never have very high protein intake as that would increase your risk of getting kicked out of ketosis as the body starts converting excess protein into glucose. However, it is also important that you consume protein in moderate quantity as, in its absence, the body can start converting lean muscle mass into glucose.

Consume plant-based protein in moderate quantity, and your protein intake should remain between 20-25% of your total calorie intake.

Some good protein sources are:

Tofu: It is a soy product that's low in carbs and has high protein content. It is a great protein source in a vegan-keto diet. Several varieties of tofu are available in the market like the regular, firm, extra firm, fermented, smoked, and silken ones. It can be used to bring variety to the food.

It is a rich source of essential amino acids, vitamins, and minerals like iron, calcium, manganese, selenium, copper, magnesium, zinc, and vitamin B1.

Tempeh: It is a fermented soy product that's high in protein, fiber, vitamins, and minerals. It helps your body maintain its muscle mass. It is rich in some important minerals like iron, calcium, niacin, magnesium, phosphorus, and manganese. It is very easy to digest and has beneficial gut bacteria too.

Edamame: It is high in protein and also has important vitamins like B6, K1, and vitamin C. You can also get minerals like iron, zinc, and calcium from it.

Mung Bean Sprouts: These sprouts are rich in protein and other nutrients like vitamin K, B, and C. It also provides you a lot of iron. Unlike other legumes, these sprouts are not high in their carb content and hence can be used in a keto diet.

Amazing Health Benefits That Await You With Keto-Vegan Diet

Super Energy Boost

Keto vegan diet is a great combo of clean energy. It helps your body source clean fuel from healthy products. Through this diet, you can completely transform the way you have been eating until now. You'll have a better understanding of food, and you'd never feel dull or lethargic. As soon as your body gets into ketosis through this diet, you will have plenty of energy to use.

The good things you eat in your keto-vegan diet would have an even greater positive impact as you'd be bypassing the side-effected in the body created by animal-based products.

Lower Risk of Heart Diseases

Keto diet starts using cholesterol and triglycerides as the main fuel, and hence the things that had been causing blockages all of a sudden become useful. This lowers the danger to your heart. Vegan diet, on the other hand, helps in increased intake of antioxidants that lower the risk of chronic inflammations that cause damage to the heart. Better insulin sensitivity created by the keto diet also helps in lowering the risk of heart diseases. In this way, the heart gets help from many corners.

Improved Cognitive Function

The keto diet was originally devised for improving cognitive function. The ketones can help in preventing cognitive damage and promote brain health. In fact, there are several neurodegenerative disorders that are being treated through a keto diet. The impact of keto diets on epilepsy, Alzheimer's, and other such diseases is a great matter of interest for the whole world. So, if you want to improve your cognitive function, reduce your carb and sugar intake, and focus on inducing ketosis.

Better Protection from Diabetes

Diabetes is a big scare. However, the keto diet can help in lowering the risk of diabetes. It improves insulin sensitivity in your body, and hence your body is able to process sugar more effectively. Diabetes is generally a result of prolonged insulin resistance in the body. When your body becomes highly exposed to sugar, it stops responding actively to insulin signals sent for glucose absorption. The longer this problem persists, the poorer sugar management will get, and this finally leads to diabetes. The ketogenic diet cuts off the glucose supply for long periods, and hence your body becomes more sensitive to insulin signals. If you are at a higher risk of diabetes, the keto diet can solve your problems to a great extent.

Ease of Maintaining Healthy Weight

Maintaining a healthy weight remains a great challenge for most people. Vegans face this challenge as their diets ultimately remain carbohydrate rich in spite of being plant-based. Ketogenic diet followers also have the risk of healthy weight management as the keto diets cannot be followed for the whole life, and you need to have breaks. During these periods of breaks, people can witness a significant rise in their weight due to improved insulin sensitivity. If you are a vegan and you follow keto diets in the stretch, you can avoid this problem completely. You learn the ways to lead a healthy life with low-carb food, and because your diet is rich in leafy greens and other plant-based products, even after you get off a keto diet, you wouldn't see a phenomenal rise in your weight. Managing your current weight would be comparatively easy for you.

Help in Fighting Cancer

Keto diets have proven their worth in fighting cancer. It has been scientifically proven that cancer cells cannot survive on fat fuel, and they only need glucose for their survival. If you go on a keto diet, you can effectively starve the cancer cells completely. This is something no medicine can do as it is very difficult to specifically target cancer cells without affecting healthy cells in that area. However, by following a keto diet, you can simply starve the cancer cells and slow the progression of cancer in the body.

Better Eyesight

The keto-vegan diet has a positive impact on the retina of your eyes. It helps in strengthening the vessels carrying blood to the eyes, and your eye health can improve remarkably. The nutrients in the vegan diet also help in strengthening your eyesight, and hence you get support from two fronts.

Anti-aging Effect

Both the keto diet and veganism promote the anti-aging effect. They help in fighting chronic inflammations that stop the signs of early aging. The high amount of clean energy in the body also promotes the formation of healthy cells that stop those signs.

Change Your Perspective- Stop Looking at Keto-Vegan Diet as a Limiting Option

When most people think of keto-vegan diets or even either of these diets separately, they are simply wondering about the limitations. This is a negative approach that would make success difficult. These aren't simply limited period diet plans but life choices. If you seal yourself in boxes, sooner or later, the feeling of claustrophobia would arise.

The better way to look at this diet is to try to find possibilities of exploring interesting meal ideas. A positive approach towards this diet would keep you motivated. These diets simply remove sugar and refined carbs from your diet. Going vegan is a personal choice that has its own positive impact on your health and mindset. If you look at the positive aspects of this diet, following it successfully in the long-term would become easier for you.

Try to Derive All Your Carbs from Non-Starchy Leafy Greens

Carbs are not good for your health. Not only from the perspective of the keto diet but also in general, carbs are a reason for unnecessary weight gain and cause a lot of health issues. High consumption of carbs would always pose a risk of pushing you out of ketosis. If you want to avoid the process of continuously counting carbs and calories, it would be best to take all your carbs from non-starchy leafy greens.

If you are consuming all or most of your carbs from non-starchy leafy greens, there will be no reason to count calories. Leafy greens are full of fiber and have negligible calories. You can have as many leafy greens as you want and wouldn't have to think about carbs.

Explore the Countless Possibilities in Protein-Rich Foods like Tofu and Tempeh

Protein is an important part of the diet, and leaving it out can be harmful. The keto-vegan diet gives you a healthy option of getting your protein fix from alternatives like tofu and tempeh. They are rich in protein and also provide essential vitamins and minerals. There is a great variety in these protein options, and you can make your meals tastier by using them. Try to explore new recipes that bring newness and taste.

Meal Planning is Essential for Success

We all are living very hectic lives. If we don't prepare well in advance, even simple meals become a herculean task. When it comes to keto-vegan diet, things can get a little more complicated as it is difficult to find quick-fixes for your hunger. The best way to deal with this problem is to plan your meals in advance. This helps you in saving time, money, and extra calories. It is very easy to plan your meals well in advance. This would save a lot of trouble, and you would feel more organized and assured. Meal planning also ensures that you have your meals ready well in advance whenever you feel hungry, and hence you wouldn't have to think of doing anything in haste.

Get Rid of Unwanted Food Items

Temptations are hard to avoid, and once you have something appealing in front of you, cheating starts to look a very attractive option. If you really want to give good health a genuine try, it is important that you get rid of all the unwanted food items from your kitchen. Unavailability is the best way to avoid all kinds of temptations. Raid your kitchen and refrigerator before beginning the keto-vegan diet and get rid of all the unwanted food items like cereals, chips, cookies, candies or other such sugar-laden card rich items. Restock your kitchen with healthier food alternatives and keep your fridge stocked with prepared meals so that you don't feel tempted to try something unhealthy.

Healthy Fats are Important

Fats are the backbone of a keto diet, but unhealthy fats will do very little to contribute to your success story. It is important that you choose your fats in a prudent manner. Include healthy fats in your diet so that ketosis can kick in fast and work effectively in bringing down your weight and fat. Unhealthy fats would only pile up in your body and wouldn't do anything good for you.

Transition Slowly

The keto-vegan transition can be tough for most people. There is no doubt that you'd have to train your body and mind to this transition. The best way to do it is to move slowly. Slow and steady wins the race should be your motto as you are trying to completely transform the way your body processes energy. If you try to do this in haste, the chances of failure will increase. Give your body some time to adjust and take baby steps in adapting to the new lifestyle.

Watch Out for Nutrient Deficiencies

Nutrient deficiencies are possible, and there is always a risk of running into them. It is very important to be watchful of nutrient deficiencies, and you must take nutrient supplements whenever necessary so that you don't face the risk of poor health.

Chapter 4: Meal Prepping- Most Significant Step toward Successful Keto-Vegan Diet

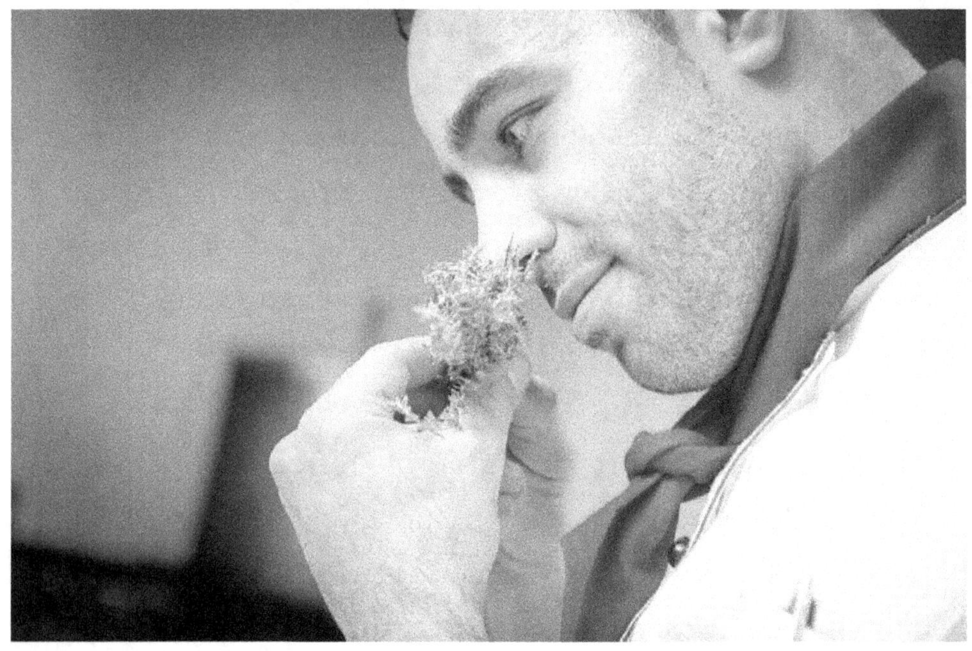

The Wonderful Concept of Meal Prepping

Necessity is the mother of inventions, and it fits even on the concept of meal prepping. There is no doubt that meal prepping is a fairly new concept.

The concept of meal prepping is a result of three important things:

1. Shortage of time to prepare meals every day
2. The need to have ready to eat food at your disposal
3. The need to have specifically prepared meals that fit our dietary requirements

This is a very fast-paced age. We all have a hectic lifestyle, and finding time to prepare meals twice or thrice a day isn't possible. In fact, most people may find it difficult to take out time every day to prepare food even once a day. Add to this, specific dietary requirements and the task would become even more challenging.

The need to have food whenever you needed gave rise to the fast-food industry. However, people have realized that fast-food isn't a healthy food option. There is very little discretion when it comes to fast food, and no matter the number of customizations the fast-food chains offer, their food would remain unhealthy due to the ingredients used.

If you have special dietary requirements or you are following any specific diet plan, then it becomes all the more difficult to rely on fast-food joints. The same goes for restaurants and diners. These are commercial establishments, and making food tastier is their primary need, and, in this process, health gets left behind.

All these factors have given rise to obesity.

People now understand the dangers of relying on fast-food, although it is still an easy, affordable, and fast option. But they still have time as a priced commodity, and hence, cooking daily isn't a viable option.

Meal prepping gives you an easy way out of this problem. In fact, it solves the complete problem in one go.

You will only need to take out a couple of hours once a week, and you can prepare and store planned meals for the whole week. Preparing in bulk not only saves time but it also saves a lot of money. Besides, you will have complete control over the ingredients, the portion size, and the number of calories you want to consume in each meal. You will have all the options for customization.

All it takes is a little bit of planning and times once a week. The food can be stored properly, and when you take it out, you'll know the exact time when it was prepared and the time till which it can go without turning bad.

The concept of meal prepping has emerged as a boon for the people who have been following any kind of specific diet plan as they can easily avoid consuming extra calories or unwanted food items. It is an economical and easy way to stay fit and healthy. During the whole week, you can simply take out a portion of food, heat it, thaw it, or refresh it, and it would be ready to eat. This convenience had given a ray of hope to all those people who were getting fed up with staring at their friends when they ate outside but couldn't eat themselves due to dietary restrictions. All those people who have very hectic weeks can simply relax when they come home as they'd know that tasty and healthy meal is waiting for them in the fridge and it'd just take few minutes to get it ready. Meal prepping makes life as simple as that.

Many people also relied on packaged food available at convenience stores. However, ready-made food is highly processed, which is very unhealthy and unfit for a person following any kind of diet. Secondly, such food packets have lots of sugar, preservatives, and trans-fat to extend its shelf life. This makes them very unhealthy.

On the contrary, meal prepping can be done consciously as per the healthy lifespan of the food items. You can also ensure that every ingredient is fresh so that you get some extra shelf life. You very well know the time for which you are preparing the food, and hence, a conscious decision can be made about the nutritiousness of the food, and you'd know for sure that you haven't been deceived.

Preparing a meal every day or having to make a decision as to the things you want to eat that day not only takes time but also cause unnecessary decision fatigue. You spend extra time and energy pondering over this insignificant thing every day, and the risk of temptations also increases several folds. If there is already a meal sitting in your bad or your fridge, you wouldn't be troubling yourself with all such questions.

All these factors make meal prepping an amazing technique that can give you immense control over your diet and would also allow you a lot of extra time.

The following chapters will explain the specific advantages of meal prepping. The techniques which can be used for meal prepping. Specific meal ideas for a whole month so that you can simply relax and let the keto-vegan diet do its job.

Helpful in Following a Specific Diet Plan

Irrespective of the type of diet plan you are following, if you are following a diet plan, eating out is insensible. The kind of food choices available always puts you at risk of crossing the calorie limit of breaching the nutritional limitations. You can never have complete control over your diet while eating out, and that's why dieters have always dreading eating out. Meal prepping has given all such people a ray of hope as they can now easily remain in calorie limits and eat only the things they want.

Saves Shopping Time and Hassle

Meal prepping means buying and preparing meals in bulk. This means you can also save money on your purchases as you would by buying things in bulk. You wouldn't have to run to the stores every now and then for restocking your supplies, and hence that also contributes towards saving time and trouble.

Better Self-Regulation

Meal preparation also helps in the prevention of personal deviation from the path to good health. When you already have healthy food prepared and stacked for the whole week, you will feel less inclined to graze unhealthy food outside. It always runs at the back of the mind that you already have your hard work and commitment about something else. On the other hand, if you don't have your meals prepared and if you start feeling hungry and you are also feeling tired, picking up the phone and ordering something to fill up the belly starts looking a lucrative option all of a sudden. To prevent such tendencies, it is better that you have prepared meals for such situations.

Waste Control

There are two parts of this, the first part is about controlling the waste that's created in packaging, and the second is about managing the wastage of food. Food packaging may not look something big but involves a lot of material, and it is all single-use. Nobody gets to reuse the food packaging, so if you have been a fan of takeaways, it adds to a lot of waste. Second, most people don't necessarily finish everything that they have ordered and bought. Bigger food portions are also responsible for this to a great extent. You haven't really put much of your hard work in the preparation process, and that also becomes a reason for the insensitivity. In all, a major portion of the food that we order gets thrown away. It is a great wastage that needs to be stopped. Meal prepping is a great way to prevent wastage. First, you reuse most of the packing material as reusable containers help in the process. Second, food wastage can be brought down to a minimum because, in one or two attempts, you really get the idea about the food portions you pack for every meal, and hence no food gets wasted.

Cost-Effective

Preparing food at home is always going to be economical, especially if you are preparing anything in bulk. However, before we prod over this, I'd like you to think about the cost of healthy prepared meals at the stores. It is way more costly than other eating options. While the junk is available at throwaway prices, you may have to shell out much more for healthy food. Preparing it at home in bulk wouldn't even cost a small amount of that. Add to this the advantage of preparing healthy and fresh food from scratch. This is an advantage you would never have when you are buying healthy food from outside if you get any. Not only this, as you buy in bulk for the whole week at least or even for a month for non-perishable goods, the cost of food goes down even further. Meal prepping can make your visits to the store economical.

Time-Saving

It is a process that requires you to work one day in a week, and for the rest of the week, you wouldn't have to focus on it. The preparation of the food once a week would take comparatively longer but not much. Compare this with preparing the meals for the whole week, and you'd find it very easy. The time you save on shopping for food several times a week or having to go out to buy food every day is huge. You save time that is spent in waiting. You also save time that you spent in figuring out the things you want to have that day. All this gets saved when you have predefined meals waiting in your fridge.

Unwinding

Having the knowledge that a major worry of the day is already taken care of can be very relaxing. We may not realize this consciously, but a part of our brain remains dedicated to the thoughts of food. It is a basic requirement, and hence it is natural for a part of the brain to remain fixated on food. The problem begins when this fixation not only starts eating our productive time and money but also causes decision fatigue. You might acknowledge that around the time of lunch, a part of your brain starts thinking about the kind of food you are going to have. It even starts analyzing the options. If you are under any type of constraint like on a diet, it may even make you feel bad and sorry. Even in the evening, after you've got free from the office if you have a burden at the back of your mind that you'll have to go and prepare the dinner, it doesn't let you be at ease. Meal prepping provides you a solution to all these problems. When you have your healthy lunch packed in your bag, there will be no reason for your brain to engage in thoughts about food. Having a set meal for the whole week also takes away the chances of decision fatigue that can be caused by thoughts of food.

Having the knowledge that every evening you can go home and relax without having to worry about cooking can be extremely relaxing, and this feeling increases, even more, when you know that the meal waiting for you is healthy and nutritious.

Meal prepping is an ideal and healthy solution for people who want to save their time and commit to a diet plan. It will take away your stress and also help you in staying in your budget. When you have ample time to plan your meals for the whole week, you feel less inclined to throw in useless alternatives and can devise ways to work with healthy food options.

To summarize, meal prepping is a healthy, affordable, and time-saving option. It is suitable for everyone. Either you have a hectic work schedule or a homemaker. If you have some extra time at your hands, you will be able to do more constructive things and contribute to your life.

Busting the Myths About Veganism and Meal Prepping

Meal prepping is a fairly new concept, and hence people have apprehensions about it. When you are already in doubt, it is very easy to spread lies or propagate myths. The same has happened even with meal-prepping, especially concerning vegan or special diets.

Here, we would discuss some common myths about meal prepping so that you can know that it is a safe, healthy, and viable alternative that can be followed without great difficulty.

Myth #1 Prepared Vegan Meals Will Lose Nutrients and Flavor

This is one of the most popular myths. However, all those people who believe in this myth never care to look at the meals they are consuming at the moment. Vegan meals would be prepared by you using fresh ingredients, and hence you will know it clearly that the food is nutritious and healthy. The processed food brought from stores has a long shelf life, and to make it that way, a lot of preservatives are added to it, compared to that vegan meal prepping is a much nutritious affair. Even the food that you buy from food chains has no surety of freshness. They also buy their ingredients in bulk, and the food may have been sitting on the shelf for much longer waiting for the customer. The thing that ensures that the food retains its flavor and nutrients is the way you package and store it. The flavor would depend on the kind of ingredients you use and the way you prepare the food. The nutrition can be preserved by correct packaging. If you wrap the food properly in aluminum foils, plastic bags, and airtight containers, it will retain its nutrient value to a great extent. If you have cooked something, ensure that it cools down before you store it in the fridge. These simple steps can help you in storing the food well easily for a week. In any case, you will be preparing a meal for about a week, and food can be stored easily for that time without the risk of getting spoiled. If you are still concerned about the freshness, be more selective while buying the ingredients and pick fruits and vegetables that are really fresh. They will add more flavor and nutrition to your food.

Myth #2 It is Difficult to Have Tasty and Healthy Options at the Same Time

There is no doubt that healthy meals may not be as tasty as fast-food as there are strong grounds for that. Most fast-food chains use salt, sugar, and tastemakers to bring that addictive flavor to the food. However, we all know how dangerous these things can be for health. Choosing veganism was the first sign that you wanted to move away from that.

However, even with vegan options, food can be made tasty. You can bring a lot of variety to your food by adding fresh and healthy alternatives. For protein, there is a great variety in tofu and tempeh. You can also add other healthy and tasty options that bring taste.

You can experiment with healthy fats like nuts, coconut, avocado to bring extra flavor in food. The leafy greens and other veggies not only add appealing color and texture to your food, but they are also very fulfilling and nutritious.

Try new dishes and find new things that can satisfy your taste buds while following the diet. Being vegan or being on a keto diet may look difficult for you, but you must not forget that a lot of people have been leading a vegan lifestyle for their whole lives. The lack of taste will only bother you as long as you keep thinking in a limited manner. Once you widen your scope of thinking, the possibilities are limitless.

Myth #3 I May Have to Eat the Same Meal Daily, It Would Get Boring

This is, again, a big myth in the minds of people. Meal planning doesn't mean that you'd have to eat the same thing daily. If that was to be the case, there wouldn't have been any need to call it meal planning. Meal planning means that you dedicate a few hours on a specific day in a week to decide the things that you'd like to eat in the day and prepare them in advance. There will be some dishes that would get repeated in the week, but they don't need to be present in every meal. You can prepare a number of things and then keep alternating them, so you have a variety. If you look closely, this is exactly what you do in your daily routine. If you go on counting the number of new things you eat in a week, the count wouldn't be very long. Here, the choice of food is going to be conscious and not forced upon you. This also means that from a list of dishes, you can also choose the dishes you like to be repeated during the week. By simply changing your perception of looking at things, you will be able to see the positive side of it more clearly.

Myth #4 Planning Meals for the Whole Week can be Tiresome

If you have been cooking regularly, then you'd know that cooking for one or cooking for 5 almost takes the same amount of time and effort. Vegan meals are generally simple and hence, don't require complex cooking processes. If you club both the things together, you will see that although preparing meals for the whole week may take some extra time one day; it isn't as complicated a process as it seems.

Myth #5 Shopping for Extensive Meal Planning Would be Exhausting

If you don't go shopping with a list, shopping can be an exhausting process. Some people feel that shopping is a relaxing activity, but most of the time, people end up buying all those things that they don't need and, in the end, feel exhausted. If you want to make your shopping experience worthwhile, prepare a complete list of things that you need to buy. Raid the specific aisle where those things are found and don't give in to the temptation of buying things that aren't on the list. Following this simple rule, you'll find that shopping even for a month is not an exhausting exercise.

Myth #6 It Would Take Up Too Much Time

Of course, cooking and packing meals for the whole week would definitely take up some time once a week. However, if you look at the time it would save during the whole week, the process would look rewarding to you. You must have a positive approach to this. If you compare it with the options you have in front of you, this would be the best thing to do.

In the first case, you simply choose to cook daily, it would definitely take up a lot more time, and the process would become taxing. This is definitely a difficult approach.

In the second case, you choose to find food outside. This will give a big setback to your healthy living option. There is no guarantee of the kind of things that would be used in the food available outside. You can't be sure of its freshness. You won't be able to achieve your health goals through such meals, and they would cost a lot.

On the other hand, meal prepping once in a week is simple and helps you in following your preferred diet plan easily. It is a cost-effective and time-saving process.

Myth #7 The Week-old Meals Would Have No Flavor

In this age of technology, this notion is flawed. We have been eating things that may have been sitting on the shelf for weeks, if not months, and we never raise a brow about them. Even the fresh fruits and vegetables that are available in the store are not fresh in the true sense, and they had been plucked long ago. We have to make do with the options available to us. Meal prepping is one of the best options if you want to save time, money, and labor. There is very little control that we have on the kind of ingredients available, meal prepping at least gives us control over the kind of nutrition we consume.

If you want to follow a keto-vegan diet, meal prepping is the best option. This can be a tough diet if you want to eat out as the number of options in front of you may be limited. You may also have no control over the portion sizes and the nutrients you get. Ultimately, following this diet plan may start getting difficult as the eating options get limited.

Meal prepping gives you variety and quality control while staying in budget.

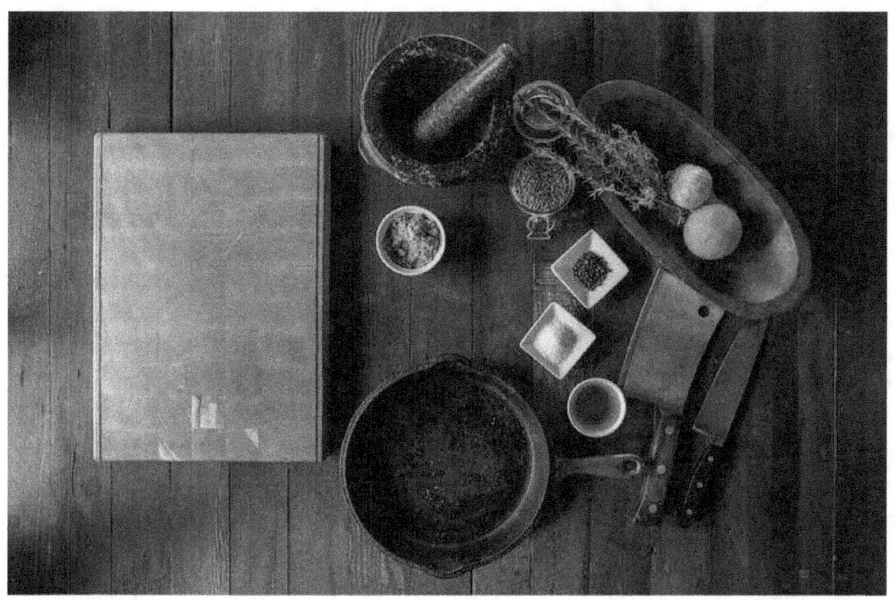

The people who had been cooking in the past find it easy to navigate the vegan lifestyle as it makes their life easier. They are used to cutting, chopping, and cooking part, and hence, the challenges in front of them are few. However, if you are not one of them, this can be a bit tough but a learning experience.

If you haven't done any cooking at all, a vegan lifestyle may still look fairly easy, as most of the recipes don't require complex cooking procedures. The major part of vegan cooking lingers around cutting and chopping. Meal prepping means that you might have to reheat your food, and hence, preparing your kitchen for that would also be a prudent option.

This part would discuss the important tools that can make your meal prepping journey easy.

Professional Knives and a Chopping Board

In vegan cooking, there is going to be a lot of cutting and chopping. You will be dealing with a lot of leafy greens, and if your cutting and chopping tools are lousy, you may face serious challenges. Invest in good quality professional knives as they make life in the kitchen simple and fast. Your chopping board should be big enough to accommodate the ingredients of at least one meal, or else there can be a lot of mess in the kitchen.

Food Processor

Food processors help in preparing salads and other things faster. You can have perfect slices of fruits and vegetables. You can also have beautifully carved veggies for salad in no time with their help. Either you want perfect zucchini spaghetti or thinly sliced cucumber that looks beautiful in your salad, perfect results can be achieved through this tool in no time. This is a good tool to have in the kitchen.

Blenders

Smoothies and protein shakes are staples, and you would need them regularly. Having a good blender would make your job easier. Invest in a blender that's heavy-duty as it would be used regularly.

Microwave

You might be preparing several meals that may need to be reheated before consuming. A hot meal is more satisfying and tasty. A microwave can help you in achieving these results easily. Microwaves provide a faster option to reheat things without loss of moisture content. If you don't have one, you can make do with your current cooking accessories, but having a microwave definitely adds speed and convenience.

Instant Pots

Instant pots are multipurpose, and they reduce your cooking time. If you don't want to invest in too many things like a slow cooker, pressure cooker, rice cooker, this simple accessory can help you with cooking faster.

All these accessories bring ease into vegan cooking, and even if you are new to cooking, they will make your life easy. Vegan cooking is comparatively simple and very healthy. You can bring a lot of variety by mixing various ingredients and inducting new alternative food items that go with your food preferences. These tools will help you in your pursuit to follow a healthy lifestyle in a more budget and time-friendly manner.

Meal Prepping Techniques

Initially, meal-prepping would require a lot of trial and error. From portion sizes to the kind of things you can have on a daily basis and the things you want to rotate, everything will have to be tested. Hence, there is no perfect start to it.

You will have to find your balance. Start with medium size portion containers and then ascertain if they are doing the job for you or not. Increase and decrease the quantity as per your needs. These adjustments will only be needed initially as with the passage of time, you'll find things getting into a routine, and you may not even need to measure things as you pack.

There are some things that you would need to keep in mind while learning the art of meal prepping. Things like deciding the size of the container, choosing the type of packing material, dealing with frozen things, and timing are a few things that may help you in this journey.

Prepare the List of Things You'd Really Like to Eat

One of the most important things for meal prepping to be successful is to find the things you can eat for the whole week. From the list of food items available, list the things you can eat more often, tabulate the things you'd like to eat on alternate days, and also write down the things you'd like to be used in most meals.

This would give you a clear picture of the number of things you'd need to prepare for the week ahead. If you want to keep it simple, keep frequently repeated things as the main course and prepare them in large batches. This would reduce your workload. Veggies that you are planning on eating regularly can be washed and trimmed so that they can be simply used in salads whenever you need them. Making a comprehensive list would make things easier, and your shopping list would also get sorted.

Find the Balance of macros

It is one of the essential steps of meal prepping. Try to find a balance of macros. Every meal portion that you prepare should be able to provide the required macros. If you want to get into ketosis, successfully ignoring this step can be a fatal mistake. People usually overlook this aspect when trying to bring flavor in their meals. One of the objectives of this exercise is to enable weight loss too.

Cut Out a Meal Plan for the Week

You must sit with a pen and paper or your computer and have a detailed look at the week ahead. Get a fair idea of the number of times you would be eating the home-made meals or if you also have plans of eating outside. Then plan the things you would like to have in breakfast, lunch, and dinner. Mark the things that you'd like to repeat and the things you'd like to use sparsely. This is definitely a time-consuming activity, but it will give you a clear picture of the week ahead. It will root out the ambiguities and would also help you in getting prepared mentally.

Prepare a Shopping List

Once you have determined the things you would like to eat in the week, it would become easy for you to prepare a shopping list. Determine the quantity of food you'd need to prepare for the week and buy highly perishable goods like fruits and vegetables in limited quantity. You can buy whole foods and fats in larger quantities as they have a comparatively longer shelf life. It'd be also wise to check if some perishable items are already present in your fridge, and they should be used first.

Prepare Common Ingredients in a Batch

There can be several ingredients that may be getting used in more than one recipe that you prepare. The best thing about planning is that you'd know about them in advance and hence you can prepare them in larger batches. This would save a lot of your time.

Buy Proper Storage Material

You not only have to prepare a whole week of food but would also need to pack them in separate containers so that it becomes as simple as picking up a packet and going. Ease of working is the name of the game here. Hence, you must have containers to pack separate meals for each day of the week.

You can use glass or steel containers or even the food-grade plastics as per your preference. However, you must ensure that the containers have caps that fit correctly as you wouldn't want them to get spoiled or contaminate other products in the fridge. Aluminum foils and plastic packs can also be used for making it easy to pack and carry the food items.

Meal Prepping Mistakes to Avoid

You Don't Need to Prepare Everything

The best thing about the vegan diet is that a big part of it includes fresh salads, fruits, and nuts. These items don't need to be prepared well in advance. Just clean, cut, and store them in separate containers, and they can be picked up and mixed to make a variety of salads. This solves a number of problems for you. First, you wouldn't have to prepare too many things. Second, your fridge wouldn't get filled with too many containers as every day you can pick some of the sorted veggies and fruits to prepare that day's salad, and it wouldn't even take a minute. This can help you in avoiding too much stress on a cooking day. When there is so much to do on a single day, even simple things like these start looking like a big task. You can avoid that by using this simple trick, and that would also ensure that there is variability in your food.

Be Careful While Freezing Things

This is important as all things can't be frozen. For instance, high moisture vegetables like tomatoes shouldn't be frozen as it would lose its shape, texture, and taste when thawed. There are several vegetables that don't work well when frozen and thawed, and hence you must do your research well.

Generally, uncooked and roasted vegetables don't thaw well. Tomato, zucchini and fresh herbs also turn up poorly when frozen and thawed.

You can freeze curries, stir-fries, soups, stews, and fried rice easily.

Avoid Incorrect Usage of Ingredients

There are some food items that don't work well when kept for long. For instance, vegetables and fruits with high iron content wouldn't turn out well when kept for long. If you try to store crispy food items with other meal preps, they might go limp or lose their structure. They don't react well to moisture. It is important to identify such things and store them separately. For instance, crispy tofu wouldn't remain crispy if you store it with other meal preps.

Don't Try to Include Too Many Complicated Things

The best way to navigate meal prep successfully is to keep things as simple as possible. You may feel the enthusiasm to stay in the kitchen for 8 hours on the first week, but as things get into a routine, you would start feeling it to be a bit taxing. The best way out is to prepare only one of two complex recipes for lunch or dinner and keep the rest simple. Mix the basic ingredients of salads and snacks and create alternate dishes.

The simpler you keep it, the easier you would find to stick to this diet plan in the long-term.

Chapter 5: Meal Planning- The Four Week Meal Planning for Keto-Vegan Success

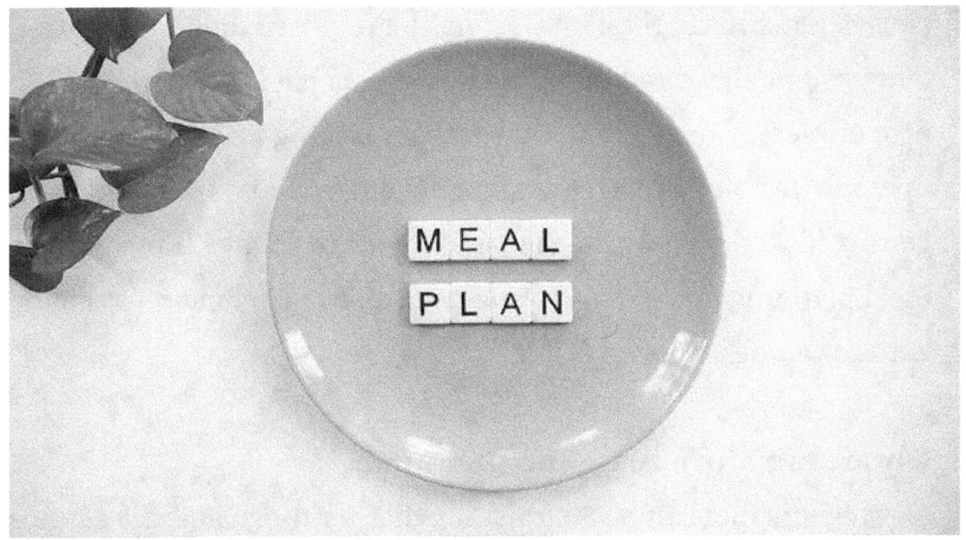

The Concept of Meal Planning

Meal planning is a crucial part that can help you in sustaining any diet correctly. It helps you in preparing the fine structure of your diet, and hence, following any diet becomes easier. Some people simply like to go with the flow, but as far as tough diets like the vegan-keto diet are concerned, meal planning can prove to be the most crucial step on the path of success.

Meal Planning Helps You in:

Entering Ketosis Faster

The ketogenic diet isn't just another fad diet but a very scientific program with intended benefits and paths. If entering ketosis is your objective, a misdirected diet may not take you anywhere, and there is a great danger of that happening in a vegan lifestyle. Veganism is a plant-based diet where exceeding carb intake always remains a problem. Getting the required amount of fat and protein also remains a question. In such a condition, if a proper meal plan is not followed, there is a high risk that you may not be able to reach the state of ketosis, or you'd keep getting kicked out of ketosis due to high carb intake. Proper meal planning helps in adopting healthier food choices so that ketosis can be achieved faster.

Obtaining More Bang for the Buck

A ketogenic diet can be a punishing diet for most, and the same can be said about a vegan lifestyle too, as both limit the number of food options in front of you. However, when you combine both, things can get really difficult. This leads to anxiety and apprehension in many people about the viability of the diet plan. If you are bearing so much trouble, you must get results better than others. Meal planning helps you in that. If you plan your meals properly, you will be consuming healthier options more, and hence the weight loss results would be much better for you.

Gives You Greater Food Choice and Variety and Customization

If you plan your meals in advance, you will not have to make last-minute compromises. You will have the time to research more recipes and find a better alternative to things you like but can't have due to diet restrictions. The option to adjust your meals as per your calorie demands is also available to you if you plan your meals in advance. This diet can get tough, and you may start feeling the pressure of limited food options. Meal planning helps you in avoiding this pressure. You will be able to bring variety in your food even with the limited options if you devote some time to planning your meals ahead of time.

Takes Away the Stress of Cooking

Cooking meals is a task many people detest, especially when they are tired or have had a long day. Meal planning can help you in taking off this stress. It gives you the chance to plan your meals, and you can prepare several different meals by mixing some common ingredient lists. This means cooking on one day of the week would ensure that you wouldn't have to cook for the rest of the week, and you can also have a variety in your meals. This becomes a very big plus point when you are stuck with a restrictive diet plan. It also helps you in avoiding the stress of daily cooking.

Makes Shopping Easy

Meal planning can make your grocery shopping really easy. You will have the list of things you'd need in the week, and hence frequent trips to the superstore for buying things can be avoided easily. It is a proven fact that shopping with a list is a more cost-effective way to shop as impulsive buying can be avoided. So, it will help you in staying in the budget.

Helps in Reducing Decision Fatigue

We have discussed this point previously, too, but it is a very important factor when it comes to food. We can spend a good amount of time trying to figure out the things we want to order or prepare. During this period, the thoughts of cheating also come once in a while, as the thoughts of food can be very tempting.

You'd find it difficult to make the things you want to eat, and the temptations to have something out of your dietary list can also become strong. Meal planning helps you in preventing both. The day you sit to plan the meals for the week, your mind is very focused, and you only include things that are permissible. You make the decisions for the whole week, and hence, for the rest of the week, there would be no decision fatigue regarding this.

Makes You More Confident

Meal planning makes you more confident about your dietary preferences. When you have planned your meals in advance, there is no uncertainty about the things you can or should eat. There is also no question about whether you will be able to meet your caloric and nutritional requirements or not. All these things are planned beforehand, and hence this makes you more confident.

Gives You Better Self Control

Avoiding temptations becomes easy as you have your meals of the day. If you don't plan your meals, controlling the mind can become really tricky.

Planning meals is not a very difficult task as you simply need to decide the things you want to eat and ensure they provide the nutrition you need. However, to make it easy, you can try the following:

Try New Apps

There are plenty of applications available online that can help you in assessing the nutritional value of the food you are planning. This helps a lot as you don't have to figure all that out all by yourself.

Include Tasty Options

Don't let your diet get boring or monotonous. There is no doubt that the task of meal prepping and meal planning is to reduce your work. Hence, you will not be preparing different meals every day. However, you can still create variations by including different ingredients in your salad. Try mixing the berries and nuts for some more taste. Throw in some tasty substitute to add flavor to your food. The more interesting your diet remains, the greater would be its chances of success.

Take the Help of Your Family and Loved Ones

Sometimes it can get too much too do everything by yourself. Managing a strict diet all by yourself while others are enjoying all kinds of meals carefreely can also start looking like a punishment. It can break your confidence and control. The best way is to discuss this with your friends and family openly. A little bit of consideration from others can make the journey easy.

Have Some Quick Solutions Ready

There can be times when you don't find the time to fix yourself the decided meals. This can happen with anyone, and you must remain prepared for it. The best way to deal with such situations is to have some keto-friendly snacks ready. You must keep something like that in your bag, too, as cravings can arise anytime. Many times, we start feeling hungry by simply looking at others who are eating. These cravings can get very strong, and this may lead to deviation from the diet plan. The presence of healthy snacks in your bag helps in preventing any such thing.

1st Week Meal Plan

	Breakfast	Lunch	Dinner
Monday	Vanilla Protein Shake with 1 Scoop of Whey Protein and 2 teaspoon	Creamy Broccoli Soup	Roasted Eggplant with Miso Tofu

	Coconut Oil		
Tuesday	Tofu Frittata	Kale Salad with Tomatoes and Walnuts	Mushroom Steaks with Avocado Chimichurri
Wednesday	Vanilla Protein Powder Shake with Coconut Milk	Creamy Broccoli Soup	Roasted Eggplant with Miso Tofu
Thursday	Tofu Frittata	Zucchini in Avocado Sauce	Cauliflower Fried Rice
Friday	High Protein Oatmeal	Kale Salad with Avocado and Berries	Mushroom Steaks with Avocado Chimichurri
Saturday	Lemon Chia Pudding	Creamy Broccoli Soup	Cauliflower Fried Rice
Sunday	High Protein Oatmeal	Zucchini in Avocado Sauce	Roasted Brussels Sprouts with Vegan Cheese

	Breakfast	Lunch	Dinner
Monday	Turmeric Coffee with Cocoa Butter	Vegetable Soup made from Vegetable Broth, Vegan Cheese and Mushroom	Tofu Kebabs
Tuesday	Tofu Scramble with Vegetables	Tofu Casserole with Broccoli	Cabbage Lasagna
Wednesday	Turmeric Coffee with Cocoa Butter	Vegetable Soup made from Vegetable Broth, Vegan Cheese and Mushroom	Zucchini Bolognese
Thursday	Tofu Scramble with Vegetables	Tofu Casserole with Broccoli	Roasted Eggplant with Miso Tofu
Friday	Bulletproof Coffee	Stir-Fried Tofu and Cauliflower	Cabbage Lasagna
Saturday	Green Protein Smoothie	Vegetable Soup made from Vegetable	Zucchini Bolognese

| | | Broth, Vegan Cheese and Mushroom | |
| Sunday | Bulletproof Coffee | Stir-Fried Tofu and Cauliflower | Cabbage Lasagna |

3rd Week Meal Plan

	Breakfast	Lunch	Dinner
Monday	Coconut Flour Waffles	Creamy Broccoli Soup	Tofu with Vegan Cheese and Mixed Greens
Tuesday	Chocolate Raspberry Chia Seed Puddings	Tofu with Cucumber and Avocado Salad	Roasted Vegetable Masala
Wednesday	Coconut Flour Waffles	Blueberry Protein Shake	Zucchini Lasagna
Thursday	Tofu Scramble with Vegetables	Creamy Broccoli Soup	Tofu with Vegan Cheese and Mixed Greens
Friday	Chocolate	Blueberry	Roasted

	Raspberry Chia Seed Puddings	Protein Shake	Vegetable masala
Saturday	Chia and Hemp Seed Oatmeal	Creamy Broccoli Soup	Zucchini Lasagna
Sunday	Coconut Flour Waffles	Tofu with Cucumber and Avocado Salad	Tofu Kebabs

4th Week Meal Plan

	Breakfast	Lunch	Dinner
Monday	Chia Pudding	Tofu Casserole with Broccoli	Smashed Bean Sandwiches
Tuesday	Coconut Flour Waffles	Kale Stew	Zucchini Alfredo
Wednesday	Coconut Yogurt Bowl	Stuffed Mushroom with Swiss Chards and Nuts	Roasted Mushroom Medley
Thursday	Turmeric Coffee with Cocoa Butter	Zucchini in Avocado Sauce	Smashed Bean Sandwiches

Friday	Coconut Yogurt Bowl	Tofu Casserole with Broccoli	Roasted Mushroom Medley
Saturday	Green Protein Smoothie	Zucchini in Avocado Sauce	Zucchini Alfredo
Sunday	Coconut Yogurt Bowl	Stuffed Mushroom with Swiss Chards and Nuts	Roasted Mushroom Medley

Ways to Maintain the Lost Weight after 28 Days of Keto-Vegan Meal Plan

Why Keto Diet is Time-Bound

Keto is a good way to bring down your fat and provide a healthy break to your body. However, as all good things must come to an end, the keto should also be done in intervals. There are several reasons for this. Although running on fat fuel is good for our body, total and longer carb deprivation can also have an unhealthy impact on the body.

Although keto helps in bringing down cholesterol in your body and improves your lipid profile, remaining in keto for very long can even create problems with your lipid profile.

There may be several other problems that you may face like:

There can be nutritional deficiencies

There are several carbs that provide essential minerals to the body, and in their prolonged absence, you can start facing health challenges. To get all the required vitamins, minerals, antioxidants, and phytochemicals that your intake of carbs remains normal and healthy. Therefore, after a certain period, you must get off your keto diet.

You may develop constipation

Certain carbs and the fibers found in them are essential for keeping your gut healthy. Following a vegan-keto lifestyle, although your fiber intake remains good, there are certain carbs that you aren't able to consume like grains. This can cause constipation. Following this diet periodically can help in getting the best of both the worlds.

Staying fit may become a challenge

Exercise plays an important role in keeping our body fit and in shape. However, while you are on keto, high-intensity interval training becomes a challenge as your carb intake goes down. This can have an impact on your physique.

There can be hormonal imbalance too

A long-term keto diet can have an adverse impact on your hormones too. For instance, thyroid production goes down. It can also lower the production of testosterone and progesterone in men and women, respectively. Hence, it isn't advisable for the long-term.

You may experience the following on getting off keto:
You May Feel Your Blood Sugar Levels Fluctuating

This is very common. It happens with almost everyone getting off keto. The reason is simple. Your carb intake on keto is very long, and hence you develop a stronger insulin sensitivity, which is a good this in itself. However, this also means that even a small amount of carb would get absorbed much quickly. Your blood sugar levels would rise suddenly after food intake and get low very soon. Although this isn't dangerous, if you follow a healthy lifestyle, it is important to remain careful about it. While on keto, there is seldom such a response and hence your body gets out of practice.

You May also Experience a Certain Amount of Weight Gain

This sometimes scares people. When you get off keto, your carb intake increases, and along with it the body also starts gaining a little bit of water weight. If you maintain a healthy lifestyle, this increase would be minimal, and you shouldn't have to bother about it. However, if you start dumping a lot of sugar or empty calories into your body, this water weight can increase alarmingly. So, if you experience some weight gain after keto, there is nothing to get alarmed of.

You May Start Feeling More Energetic

The carbs get absorbed more quickly and hence give you an energy kick. This doesn't happen on keto as your energy levels remain constant. With increased carb intake, you will feel your energy levels suddenly going up and down. Mind the kind of carbs you are consuming if you want to maintain stability.

You Can Also Experience Bloating

Reintroduction of certain fiber-rich food can cause bloating in the beginning. You don't need to get alarmed by it. The bloating is a temporary phenomenon and would go away very soon as your gut gets accustomed to new food items.

Your Appetite May Go Up

This is a significant change people may experience after getting off keto. People think that this happens due to boring keto food. The lower appetite in keto is a result of energy abundance and lower dependence on food for energy. The body is in ketosis, and hence it is actually burning your body fat for producing energy. That's why you don't feel very hungry on a keto diet. However, that changes when you start a high-carb diet. A high carb diet increases your blood glucose levels fast, but it gets used up very quickly, and hence, you start feeling hungry very often. This doesn't have anything to do with the taste of food. So, if your appetite goes up after getting off a keto diet you must know that it is a normal process. However, if you are feeling hungry very often you do need to watch your diet. It happens when you are consuming a very high-carb diet or empty calories, and that's unadvisable by all standards.

The Important Things to Keep in Mind While Getting Off a Ketogenic Diet

It is very important that you remain careful when you get off your keto diet as carelessness can cause weight relapse. There are some very simple things which, if not kept in mind, can also pose health risks. If you want to maintain your lost weight, you must keep in mind the following things:

It is Important to Keep Carbs Low and Fiber High-Increase Your Carb Intake Slowly

Quality of carbs that you consume matters a lot when you get off your keto diet. If you start consuming a lot of refined carbs or empty calories, your body may react adversely. Being on keto means that your body's exposure to carbs goes down considerably. Therefore, the carbs should be reintroduced slowly.

Most of the carbs that you consume must come from vegetables. You can include the starchy vegetables too in your diet. However, you must stay away from refined carbs and completely away from refined sugar.

Every gram of carb would also add four grams of water to your system. If your carb intake goes up significantly, you may even experience a steep weight increase.

The best way to get off a keto diet is to follow a Mediterranean diet. Include as much as vegetables and fresh foods in your diet, and you would be able to prevent weight gain to a great extent. The carb intake would have to be increased as you have been taking very few carbs in keto. But you must not increase it all of a sudden. Ensure that the carb increment is gradual from all your food sources.

The higher the amount of fiber in your food, the easier it would become for your body to adapt to the change as fiber helps in better management of blood glucose levels, and hence it would also help you in managing your weight successfully.

Slightly Increase the Amount of Lean Protein Intake
When you get off your keto diet, your fat intake will become low, and carb intake would become high. However, the more you consume carb, the faster would be the weight gain. The best way to deal with this problem is to slightly increase your protein intake too. The conversion of protein into calories is a tedious process, and it consumes more energy in the process. Hence,

you will be able to burn more calories in this way. Vegans can get lean protein through many sources, and hence it is a very easy task for them. In fact, most of the legumes that were off-limits in keto would be available now, and they have good amounts of carbs and fiber too. Increasing the intake of legumes can do the trick for you, and it would get easier to manage weight.

Keep a Diet Plan in Mind- Don't Let Your Guard Down
The biggest reason for weight relapse after people get off diets is their carelessness and binge eating. They start eating all those things in large quantities that weren't permitted. This leads to a meteoric weight rise. If you want to manage your weight successfully, you must ensure that you don't start binge eating carbs, especially things that are rich in refined sugar.

In the Beginning, Consume Only Unprocessed Carbs
This is also a very important thing if you want to manage your weight successfully. You must not consume processed food in high quantities as it contains a lot of sugar. These are full of refined carbs and sugar and would cause a lot of problems for your system. It would also lead to blood sugar level fluctuations and food cravings. This would also increase your food intake, and hence weight gain can take place.

Your Portion Sizes Must Remain Limited

Initially, you must watch your food portions very carefully. While having carbs, it is very easy to consume more carbs as your frequency of meals may also increase. This is not very healthy and definitely bad for weight control. You must watch your frequency of meals as well as the size of your portions. In fact, you must start with smaller meal sizes and then increase them gradually as per need.

Give Your Body the Transition Time

Last but not least, give your body the time to adjust to this change. The transition to keto wasn't easy for the body, and transition from keto to carb-rich diet would also not be easy. It would also require a complete switch over of the fuel supply mechanism. The longer you give to your body to adjust to the change, the easier and better it would be for you. You must never try to bring any change in haste. Give your body the transition time, and you will be able to manage your weight more effectively and would have the least side effects. Managing weight is one of the biggest challenges that people face when they get off any diet. Most of the reasons for that have been explained here so that you don't have to face weight relapse. Good health depends a lot on our healthy lifestyle choices and the discipline we show in our personal lives. Most people think that simply by following a certain diet, they can have a healthy body. They are highly mistaken as gradually these steps stop showing results if we don't follow a disciplined life. Showing restraint is very important, and that's one thing that can take you a long way on your weight loss journey. If you want to maintain your lost weight, simply stick to a healthy lifestyle and maintain a safe distance from simple carbs or refined carbs. Eat as much natural as possible and avoid highly processed food irrespective of the fact that it comes in the grab of being vegan. These simple steps can help you in staying healthy and fit for very long.

Conclusion

Thank you for making it through to the end of this book, let's hope it was informative and able to provide you with all of the tools you need to achieve your goals whatever they may be.

Keto and vegan lifestyle have their own independent fan following. Both of these methods have been used by people to get weight loss and health benefits.

Ketogenic lifestyle is a proper diet to help weight loss and get several health benefits. It was designed by doctors while treating patients suffering from neurological issues, and it was found to be very effective. Later on, the doctors also realized its use in helping people lose weight. It is a diet plan that enforces some dietary restrictions but has shown definite results.

On the other hand, veganism is more of a lifestyle choice than a diet plan. It is a way of life. It is for the people who feel for the animals and want to follow a diet that doesn't involve animal meat or animal products. It a very environmentally sensitive diet. These days more and more people are following this diet also for its health benefits, especially weight loss.

This diet relies more on leafy greens and low potency items, and hence, managing weight becomes easier in this dietary system.

A keto vegan diet is a marriage of both the worlds. It can help you in incorporating the benefits of both the lifestyles.

This book has tried to explain the basics of both the lifestyles and the ways in which they can be used together. This book has discussed the things where you will have to reach a compromise and also the places where you'll feel that they are very liberal.

This book also discusses two other very important things that can play a very role in the success of a keto-vegan lifestyle. Those things are meal prepping and meal planning.

You have read that meal prepping can prove to be a stepping stone to success as you get to follow this lifestyle with ease. Whereas meal planning would help you in assessing the flow of your week as well as the kind of ingredients you would be consuming. Remember, the objective of this diet is to bring weight loss and other health benefits.

This book will help you in understanding these basics so that you are able to achieve your goals successfully.

You can also get all the benefits of the process by following the simple steps given in the book. I hope that this book is really able to help you in achieving your goals.

Finally, if you found this book useful in any way, a review on Amazon is always appreciated!

www.ingramcontent.com/pod-product-compliance
Lightning Source LLC
Chambersburg PA
CBHW061750250726
48657CB00001B/60